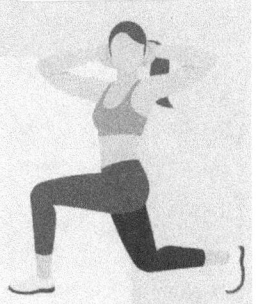

WALL PILATES WORKOUTS FOR WOMEN

Wall Pilates Workouts for Women: 28-Day Challenge to Sculpt Your Strong & Confident Body - Complete Illustrated Step-by-Step Exercises for Perfect Posture, Strength, Balance, Boost Energy & Reduce Stress

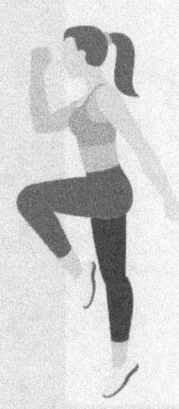

CHLOE TONKIN

TABLE OF CONTENTS

TABLE OF CONTENTS 2

WELCOME MESSAGE 7

CHAPTER 1 - INTRODUCTION.. 8

MY JOURNEY WITH WALL PILATES... 8

YOUR NEW FITNESS ALLY: WHY WALL PILATES WILL CHANGE YOUR LIFE 9

PHYSICAL, MENTAL, AND EMOTIONAL ADVANTAGES FOR WOMEN 9

CHAPTER 2 - FOUNDATIONS OF WALL PILATES 10

THE CORE PRINCIPLES OF PILATES & WALL ADAPTATION............................ 10

CHAPTER 3 - YOUR PILATES TOOLKIT 11

NECESSARY TOOLS AND ACCESSORIES FOR EFFECTIVE WALL PILATES WORKOUTS . 11

SETTING UP YOUR PILATES SPACE... 12

TIPS ON MAINTAINING PROPER FORM AND PREVENTING INJURIES 13

PROPER ALIGNMENT CHECK 14

CHAPTER 4 - WARM-UP AND COOLING DOWN................................ 16

WARM-UP: PRELIMINARY EXERCISES.. 16

NECK STRETCHES.. 16

ARM CIRCLES... 18

WALL LEG SWINGS.. 19

WALL ROLL DOWN.. 21

SHOULDER ROLLS... 22

WALL HIP CIRCLES.. 24

WALL SQUATS.. 27

ANKLE CIRCLES 28

COOLING DOWN: THE ESSENTIAL WIND-DOWN 30

CHAPTER 5 - CORE EXERCISES: SCULPT & STRENGTHEN YOUR CORE.......... 32

WALL MOUNTAIN CLIMBERS 32

ISOMETRIC WALL PLANK HOLD 34

WALL LEG RAISES 35

WALL OBLIQUE CRUNCHES 37

VERTICAL WALL SIT & TWIST 39

WALL DEAD BUG 40

WALL SIDE PLANK 43

HIGH WALL KNEE TUCKS (INVERTED) 45

CHAPTER 6 - UPPER BODY EXERCISES: TONE & DEFINE YOUR UPPER BODY 47

WALL ROW 47

WALL ROW ISOHOLD 49

HINGE TO WALL 51

WALL TRICEP EXTENSION 52

WALL ER (EXTERNAL ROTATION) 54

WALL PUSH UP PLUS 57

WALL PUSH UP 59

FLOOR PUSH UP 61

CHAPTER 7 - LOWER BODY EXERCISES: SHAPE & DEFINE YOUR LOWER BODY 64

WALL SQUAT HOLDS 64

ELEVATED WALL LUNGES 67

WALL-SUPPORTED PISTOL SQUATS 69

GLUTE BRIDGE WALL SLIDES 71

WALL SIDE LEG LIFTS 73

WALL SQUAT WITH CALF RAISE 75

ELEVATED STALLION PULSES 77

HIGH WALL GLUTE KICKBACKS 79

HIP FLEXOR MARCH 81

WALL GLUTE BRIDGE. 82

WALL FIRE HYDRANT 84

WALL COSSACK SQUAT 86

WALL-FACING SQUAT *88*

CHAPTER 8 - FLEXIBILITY & BALANCE EXERCISES **90**

FLEXIBILITY 91

WALL FORWARD FOLD *91*

WALL CHEST OPENER *93*

WALL TRICEP STRETCH *95*

WALL HIP FLEXOR STRETCH *97*

WALL QUAD STRETCH *99*

BALANCE 101

SINGLE LEG STANCE *101*

SINGLE LEG WALL STAND *102*

WALL LEG SWING *104*

WALL HEEL-TO-TOE WALK *107*

WALL BALANCE KNEE RAISES *109*

CHAPTER 9 - FUN PARTNER WORKOUTS **111**

ENGAGING EXERCISES THAT CAN BE DONE WITH A FRIEND FOR ADDED MOTIVATION

.... 111

WALL PILATES BALL PASS *111*

PARTNER WALL SQUATS *113*

WALL PLANK HIGH FIVES *115*

WALL SEATED TWIST PARTNER STRETCH *116*

CHAPTER 10 - 28-DAY CHALLENGE TO TRANSFORM YOUR BODY **119**

WEEK 1: CORE SCULPT & STRENGTHEN 119

Day 1: Foundation Day *119*

Day 2: Core Activation *119*

Day 3: Core Challenge *119*

Day 4: Recovery and Stretch *119*

Day 5: Full Core Engagement *120*

Day 6: Flexibility Focus *120*

Day 7: 120

WEEK 2: UPPER BODY TONE & DEFINE 120

Day 8: Upper Body Foundation 120

Day 9: Triceps and Chest 120

Day 10: Push and Pull 120

Day 11: Recovery and Stretch 121

Day 12: Upper Body Endurance 121

Day 13: Flexibility Focus 121

Day 14: 121

WEEK 3: LOWER BODY SHAPE & DEFINE 121

Day 15: Lower Body Foundation 121

Day 16: Glutes Activation 121

Day 17: Squats and Pulses 121

Day 18: Recovery and Stretch 122

Day 19: Full Lower Body Challenge 122

Day 20: Flexibility Focus 122

Day 21: 122

WEEK 4: BALANCE AND FLEXIBILITY 122

Day 22: Full Body Balance 122

Day 23: Walking and Balance 122

Day 24: Flexibility and Balance 122

Day 25: Recovery and Stretch 123

Day 26: Core and Balance Integration 123

Day 27: Full Body Challenge 123

Day 28: 123

CHAPTER 11 - BONUS CONTENT 124

FUEL YOUR FITNESS: ENERGIZING SMOOTHIES & BALANCED MEALS. 124

ENERGIZING SMOOTHIE RECIPES: 124

Citrus Boost Smoothie: 124

Berry Blast Antioxidant Smoothie: 125

Pineapple Mint Delight: 125

Mango Turmeric Elixir 126

Chocolate Peanut Butter Protein Shake: 126

Green Tea & Berry Fusion: 127

BALANCED MEAL IDEAS: 128

Quinoa Chickpea Buddha Bowl: 128

Salmon Avocado Quinoa Salad: 128

Mediterranean Lentil Soup: 129

Stir-Fried Tofu & Vegetable Quinoa: 129

Chicken & Avocado Wrap: 130

Sweet Potato Black Bean Chili: 130

SNACK ATTACK: 131

Trail Mix Crunch: 131

Caprese Skewers: 131

Greek Yogurt & Berry Parfait: 131

Cucumber Hummus Boats: 132

Apple Slices with Almond Butter: 132

Edamame Power Pods 133

GUIDANCE ON PERSONALIZED ROUTINES & WEEKLY SCHEDULES 133

PRINTABLE PROGRESS TRACKERS 136

WEEKLY WORKOUT PLANNER 140

CHAPTER 12 - CONCLUSION – STAY MOTIVATED **149**

LEGAL DETAILS 150

WELCOME MESSAGE

Welcome to "Wall Pilates Workouts for Women: 28-Day Challenge to Sculpt Your Strong & Confident Body." I am thrilled to embark on this transformative journey with you. Whether you're a seasoned fitness enthusiast or stepping into the world of Pilates for the first time, this book is designed to be your ultimate guide to achieving strength, flexibility, and balance through wall-based exercises.

Get ready to embrace a fitness ally that goes beyond physical benefits. Wall Pilates is not just a workout; it's a holistic approach to well-being. Together, we'll delve into exercises that sculpt and tone, enhance your mental clarity, and empower you with a newfound confidence.

This book is not just about the exercises; it's about your journey toward a healthier, more vibrant you. Let's build a foundation of strength, embrace flexibility, and foster balance that extends beyond the mat and into every aspect of your life.

Get ready to transform, inspire, and discover the power of Wall Pilates.

Welcome aboard!

CHAPTER 1 - INTRODUCTION

MY JOURNEY WITH WALL PILATES

As your guide on this Pilates journey, let me share a bit about my own experience with Wall Pilates. My reflection used to mock me - tired eyes, slumped shoulders, a stranger in my own skin. Work, motherhood, the never-ending hustle... I craved escape, not another intimidating gym or fad diet. Then, a friend, radiant and glowing, introduced me to Wall Pilates. "It's different," she promised, "gentle yet powerful, perfect for busy women like us."

I discovered the transformative power of Wall Pilates during a time when I was seeking a workout that not only challenged my body but also brought a sense of joy and mindfulness to my routine. The adaptability and effectiveness of wall-based exercises became a game-changer for me. Each exercise, simple yet deliberate, awakened muscles I didn't know existed. I wasn't pushing myself to the point of collapse, but I could feel my body working, strengthening, and thanking me for the attention.

Week after week, I continued with the routine. My posture improved, my core tightened, and my energy levels soared. But the most significant change was within. I started seeing my body not as a burden, but as a vessel of strength and resilience. It wasn't just about physical transformation; it was about rediscovering the woman beneath the exhaustion, the one who was strong, capable, and worthy of love and respect.

Through years of practice, learning, and teaching, I've seen the profound impact Wall Pilates has on women's lives, enhancing physical strength, and mental well-being, and sparking positive change.

In this book, I share the insights and exercises that fueled my journey. Whether you seek a sculpted core, improved posture, or a balanced lifestyle, join me in exploring Wall Pilates – a path to progress, not perfection. Let's embark on this transformative journey together, embracing strength, confidence, and well-being.

Stay inspired!

YOUR NEW FITNESS ALLY: WHY WALL PILATES WILL CHANGE YOUR LIFE

Hey Beautiful 🧘 💭 ✨ ,

Ever had a fitness ally that's not just a routine but a life-changer? Well, get ready to meet your new BFF: Wall Pilates. This isn't your average workout; it's a transformative journey waiting to happen.

Think of Wall Pilates as that friend who's always got your back, guiding you through movements that sculpt your body and clear your mind. It's not just about reps; it's about unlocking strength you didn't know existed, fostering flexibility that feels like freedom, and balancing your body in a way that spills over into every part of your life.

But it's more than just exercise; it's a lifestyle shift. Wall Pilates is about embracing a version of you that's strong, confident, and oh-so-vibrant. So, say goodbye to the same-old workouts and hello to a fitness adventure that's about to change your life.

Get ready to fall in love with fitness in a whole new way.

PHYSICAL, MENTAL, AND EMOTIONAL ADVANTAGES FOR WOMEN

PHYSICAL POWER:

- Sculpted core, toned limbs, and improved posture.
- Wall Pilates shapes your body for strength and confidence.
- Gentle on joints, improves mobility

MENTAL CLARITY:

- Sync your mind and body through Wall Pilates.
- Experience enhanced mental clarity and sharper focus.
- Energize yourself every day.
- Reduces stress & promotes calmness

EMOTIONAL RESILIENCE:

- Build emotional resilience through a workout that uplifts your spirits.
- Transform not just physically, but also emotionally, for a more empowered you.

CHAPTER 2 - FOUNDATIONS OF WALL PILATES

THE CORE PRINCIPLES OF PILATES & WALL ADAPTATION.

CONTROL: Pilates emphasizes controlled, precise movements that target specific muscle groups. Wall Pilates adaptations often involve holding positions or moving slowly, ensuring you engage the right muscles with maximum effectiveness.

CENTERING: Pilates revolves around strengthening your core, the powerhouse of your body. Wall Pilates exercises often utilize the wall for added stability, allowing you to focus on engaging your core muscles deeper and more effectively.

CONCENTRATION: Ever find your mind wandering during a workout? Pilates helps you stay focused. Now, think about doing that against the wall. It's like each exercise becomes a mindful journey, making your mind and body work together.

ALIGNMENT: Proper alignment is paramount in Pilates, ensuring optimal movement and preventing injury. Wall Pilates adaptations often provide visual cues and support from the wall, helping you maintain correct alignment throughout each exercise.

BREATH: Pilates emphasizes mindful breathing, using it to fuel your movements and connect with your core. Wall Pilates incorporates this seamlessly, guiding your breath with each exercise. Imagine inhaling as you lengthen your spine and exhaling as you engage your core, creating a rhythmic flow that energizes your workout.

EVERYBODY WINS: Pilates caters to all fitness levels and abilities. Wall Pilates adaptations take this inclusivity a step further. By adjusting exercises based on your needs and using the wall for support, you can tailor the workout to your unique body, ensuring a safe and effective experience.

CHAPTER 3 - YOUR PILATES TOOLKIT

NECESSARY TOOLS AND ACCESSORIES FOR EFFECTIVE WALL PILATES WORKOUTS

1. **The Essential Partner: A Sturdy Wall**

   Find a clear wall space, free from furniture or obstacles, to act as your anchor and support. Imagine it as your silent workout buddy, always there to provide stability and guidance.

2. **A Touch of Comfort (Optional): A Yoga Mat**

   While not strictly necessary, a yoga mat can provide added cushioning and comfort, especially for floor exercises or kneeling positions. Think of it as a luxurious upgrade for your workout sanctuary.

3. **A Water Bottle:**

   Staying hydrated is essential for any workout, and Wall Pilates is no exception. Keep a reusable water bottle by your side to quench your thirst and fuel your movements. Imagine taking refreshing sips as you celebrate your progress, feeling energized and revitalized.

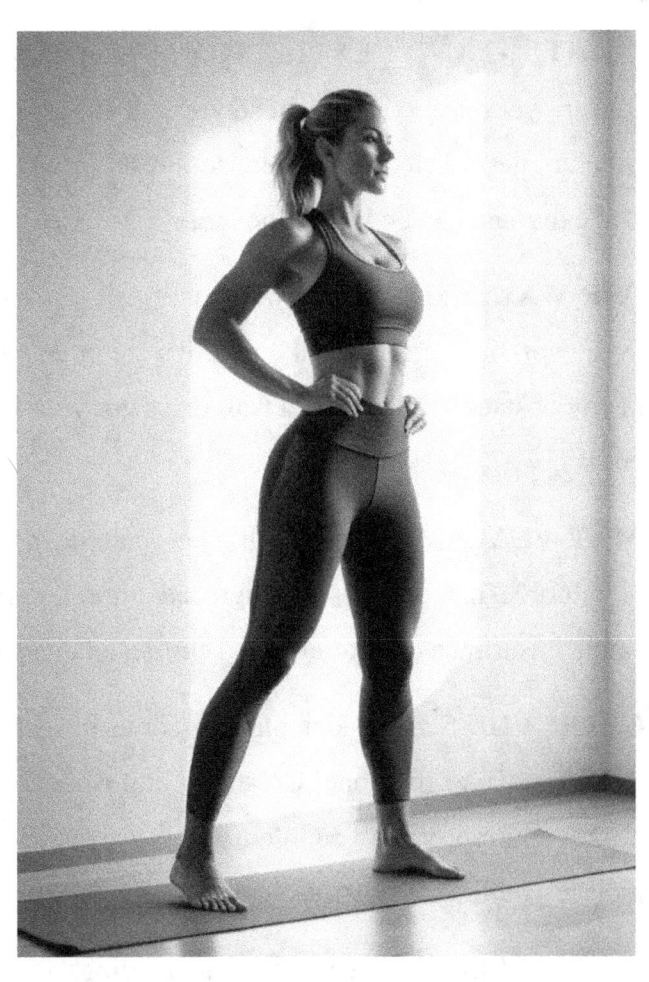

4. **Comfortable Clothing:** Choose breathable, flexible clothing that allows for unrestricted movement. Imagine feeling confident and comfortable as you move with grace and ease.

Optional Enhancements:

- **Light Weights:** Add some extra muscle-burning intensity with light weights (think 2-5 lbs) for arm exercises or weighted squats.

- **Resistance Bands:** Elevate your workout with resistance bands, adding an extra challenge to various exercises and targeting specific muscle groups.

SETTING UP YOUR PILATES SPACE

Now, let's chat about setting up the perfect space for your Wall Pilates workouts. Creating your little Pilates haven is simple, and it makes a big difference.

1. LIGHTING AND VENTILATION: Natural light is a winner, but good artificial lighting works too. Make sure your space is well-lit so you can see your movements. Ensure proper ventilation, especially if you tend to get warm during exercise. Fresh air will keep you energized and focused and can make your Pilates experience even more enjoyable.

2. THE WALL: Find a clear wall space – it's going to be your workout partner. Make sure it's clean and free from any obstacles. You want a wall that's got your back (literally).

3. MAT PLACEMENT: Unroll your mat on a flat, stable floor. This creates a designated area for your workout, ensuring a comfortable and slip-resistant space.

4. GOOD VIBES: Consider playing some music if it helps you get into the zone. Create an atmosphere that energizes and motivates you. Your Pilates space should be a place you look forward to.

5. SAFETY FIRST: Check your surroundings for any potential hazards. Make sure the floor is slip-resistant, and there's enough space for you to move around without bumping into things.

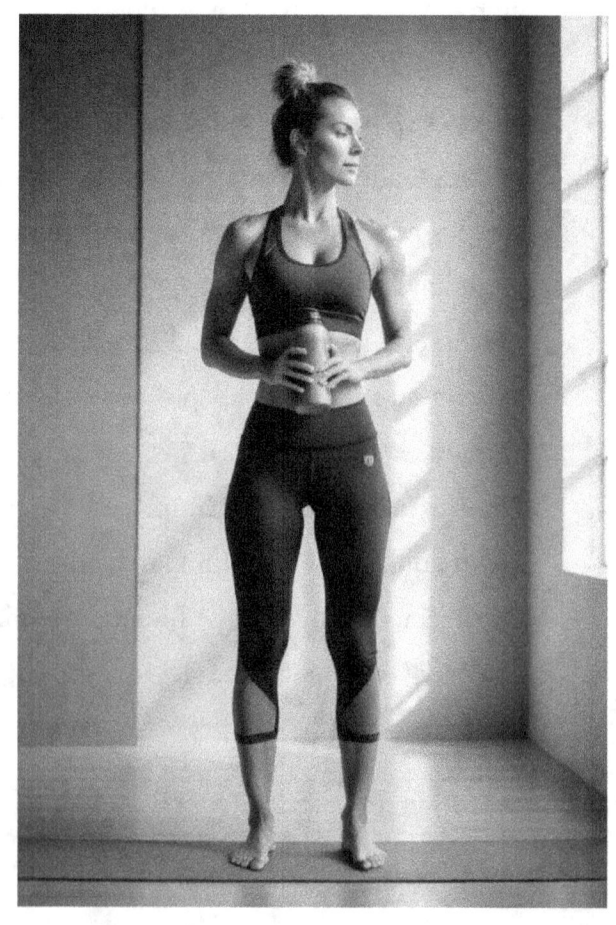

6. MOTIVATIONAL MESSAGES: Hang up inspirational quotes or images that resonate with your fitness goals. Imagine seeing them every time you step into your space, fueling your determination.

Now, take a moment to visualize your Pilates space – a well-lit, clutter-free zone with a supportive wall, your favorite mat, and all your Pilates tools ready to roll. It's not just a workout area; it's your personal Pilates haven.

TIPS ON MAINTAINING PROPER FORM AND PREVENTING INJURIES

Ensuring proper form is like giving your Pilates workout a VIP pass to effectiveness. Let's delve into some tips to maintain that impeccable form and keep injuries at bay.

1. ALIGNMENT AWARENESS:

Take a moment to check your alignment regularly. Proper alignment ensures that your muscles engage as intended, making each movement more effective.

2. CORE ENGAGEMENT:

Activate your core muscles throughout your workout. It's not just about your abs – think of your core as a stabilizing force, supporting your spine and overall posture.

3. SMOOTH TRANSITIONS:

Avoid abrupt movements between exercises. Smooth transitions help in maintaining control and reduce the risk of strain or injury.

4. LISTEN TO YOUR BODY:

Pay attention to how your body feels during each movement. If something doesn't feel right, modify the exercise or take a break. Your body knows best.

5. BREATHING RHYTHM:

Sync your breath with your movements. Proper breathing not only oxygenates your muscles but also helps in maintaining focus and control.

6. START SLOW, PROGRESS STEADY:

If you're new to Pilates or introducing a new exercise, start at a comfortable pace. Gradually increase intensity as your strength and familiarity grow.

7. QUALITY OVER QUANTITY:

Focus on the quality of your movements rather than the quantity. Precise, controlled motions are more effective and safer than rushed, haphazard ones.

9. LISTEN TO YOUR INSTRUCTOR:

Carefully follow the cues in Instructional guidance, it keeps you on the right track keeps you on the right track.

10. WARM UP AND COOL DOWN:

Never skip the warm-up or cool-down. Warming up prepares your muscles for action while cooling down helps in preventing stiffness and promotes flexibility.

Remember, Pilates is about the journey, not just the destination. By maintaining proper form and listening to your body, you're not only preventing injuries but also maximizing the benefits of your Pilates practice.

PROPER ALIGNMENT CHECK

Proper alignment is the cornerstone of a successful Pilates practice. Let's dive into the essentials of aligning your body for optimal results and a safe, effective workout.

1. HEAD POSITION: Keep your head in a neutral position, aligning it with your spine. Avoid tilting your head forward or backward. Imagine a string gently lifting you from the crown of your head.

2. SPINAL ALIGNMENT: Your spine is your Pilates' backbone. Maintain a natural curvature, ensuring each vertebra is stacked on top of the other. Picture your spine as a string of pearls – straight and aligned.

3. SHOULDER PLACEMENT: Relax your shoulders and keep them away from your ears. Engage your shoulder blades by gently pulling them down and towards each other. This promotes an open chest and proper upper body alignment.

4. HIP ALIGNMENT: Align your hips parallel to the floor. Avoid tilting or hiking your hips during exercises. A stable pelvis supports the proper engagement of the core muscles.

5. KNEE AND ANKLE ALIGNMENT: When standing or in weight-bearing positions, ensure your knees are in line with your ankles. This alignment provides stability and protects your joints from unnecessary stress.

6. FOOT POSITION: Your feet are your foundation. Keep them hip-width apart and parallel. Distribute your weight evenly across both feet, promoting stability and balance.

7. ENGAGE YOUR CORE: Activate your core muscles by drawing your navel towards your spine. This engagement not only supports your spine but also enhances the effectiveness of Pilates movements.

8. NEUTRAL PELVIC POSITION: Maintain a neutral pelvis to protect your lower back. Imagine a bowl of water on your pelvis – neither tipping forward nor spilling backward.

9. JOINT ALIGNMENT: Ensure proper alignment of joints throughout each movement. Misaligned joints can lead to discomfort and hinder the effectiveness of the exercise.

10. BODY AWARENESS: Stay mindful of your body's alignment during your entire Pilates session. Regularly check in with your posture to reinforce good habits and correct any deviations.

By incorporating these alignment checks into your Pilates routine, you're not just exercising; you're sculpting a body that moves with grace, strength, and longevity.

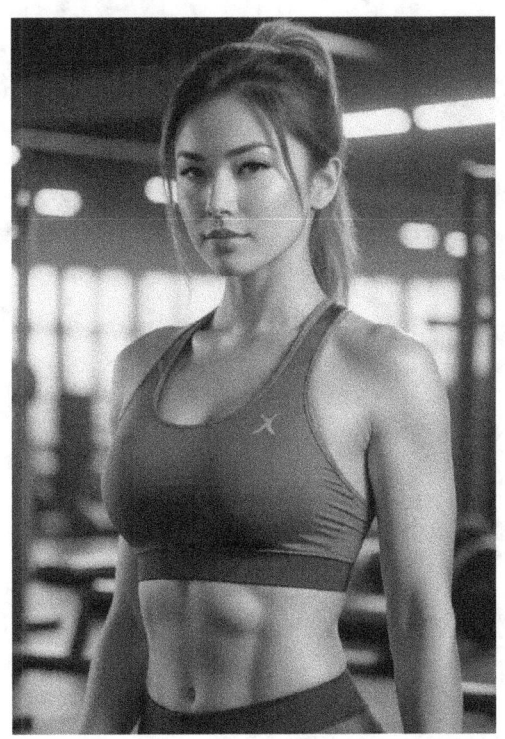

CHAPTER 4 - WARM-UP AND COOLING DOWN

WARM-UP: PRELIMINARY EXERCISES

Before we dive into the heart of your Pilates workout, let's lay the foundation with some essential warm-up exercises. Think of it as giving your body a gentle wake-up call, preparing it for the more intense movements to come.

NECK STRETCHES

1. NECK TILT SIDE TO SIDE:

Procedure:

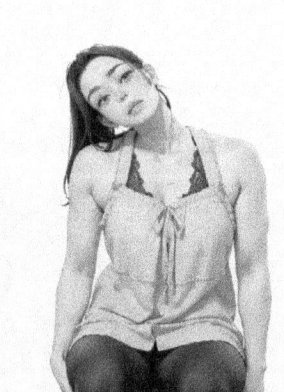
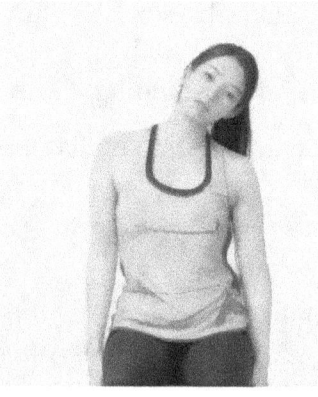

- Begin in a comfortable, seated or standing position with your spine straight.
- Slowly tilt your head to one side, bringing your ear towards your shoulder.
- Hold the stretch for 15-30 seconds, feeling a gentle stretch along the opposite side of your neck.
- Repeat on the other side.

2. NECK ROTATION:

Procedure:

- Start in the same seated or standing position with a straight spine.
- Slowly turn your head to one side, bringing your chin towards your shoulder.
- Hold the stretch for 15-30 seconds, feeling a gentle stretch in the opposite direction.
- Repeat on the other side.

3. NECK FORWARD AND BACKWARD TILT:

Procedure:

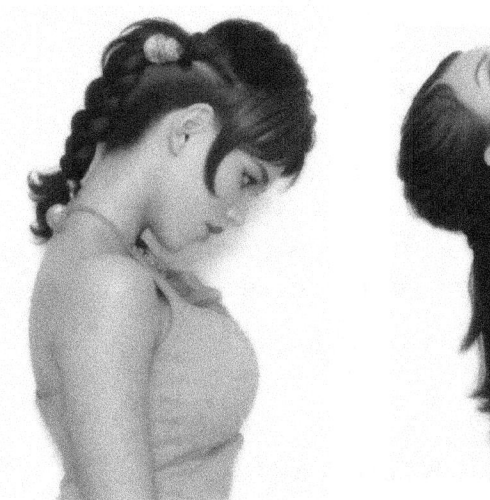

- Begin with your head in a neutral position.
- Slowly tilt your head forward, bringing your chin towards your chest.
- Hold the stretch for 15-30 seconds, feeling a stretch along the back of your neck.
- Gently tilt your head backward, looking towards the ceiling.
- Hold for 15-30 seconds, feeling a stretch along the front of your neck.

4. NECK CIRCLES:

Procedure:

- Start with a neutral head position.
- Slowly and gently rotate your head in a circular motion.
- Complete 5-10 rotations in one direction and then switch to the other direction.
- Focus on smooth, controlled movements to avoid any strain.

5. COMBINATION MOVEMENTS:

Procedure:

- Combine different neck movements, such as tilting, rotating, and circling, in a fluid sequence.
- Move within your comfortable range of motion, avoiding any abrupt or forceful movements.
- Perform these combination movements for 1-2 minutes to enhance overall neck mobility.

INSTRUCTIONAL TIPS:

- Perform neck stretches slowly and mindfully, avoiding sudden or jerky movements.
- Keep your shoulders relaxed during the stretches, allowing the focus to be on the neck muscles.
- Breathe deeply and rhythmically throughout each stretch, enhancing relaxation.

ARM CIRCLES

1. STARTING POSITION:

- Stand with your feet shoulder-width apart.
- Extend your arms out to the sides, parallel to the ground, forming a "T" shape.

2. CIRCULAR MOTION FORWARD:

- Begin by making small circles with your arms, moving them in a forward direction.
- Gradually increase the size of the circles as you warm up.

3. CIRCULAR MOTION BACKWARD:

- After completing forward circles, switch to moving your arms in a backward circular motion.
- Again, start with smaller circles and gradually increase their size.

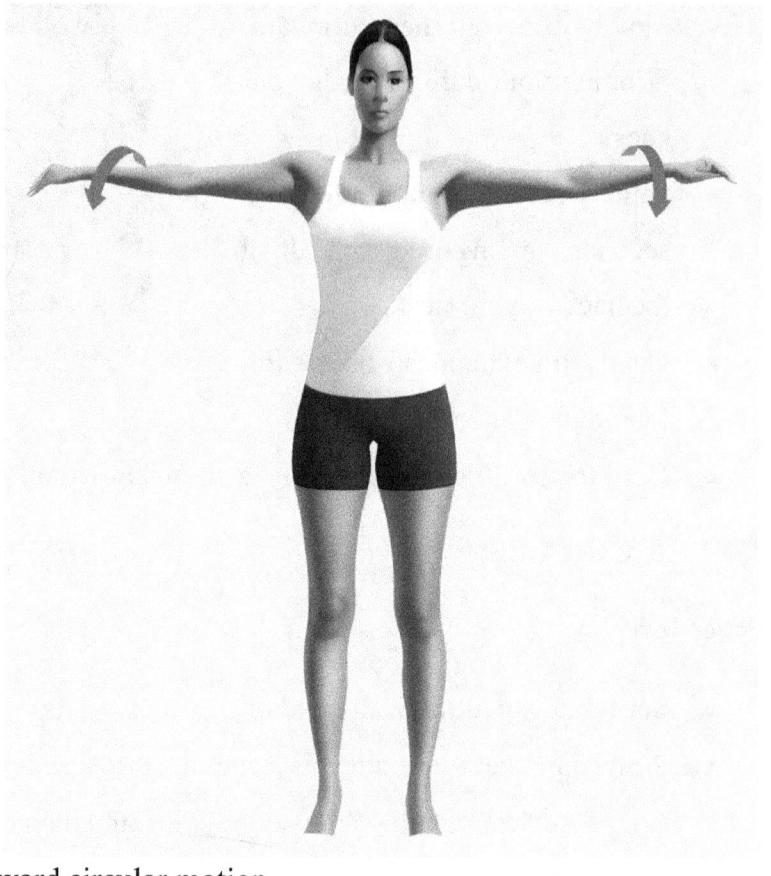

4. FOCUS ON FORM:

- Keep your shoulders relaxed throughout the movement.
- Engage your core to maintain stability.
- Ensure that your circles are controlled, avoiding rapid or jerky movements.

5. BREATHING RHYTHM:

- Inhale as your arms move upward, and exhale as they move downward.
- Sync your breath with the circular motion to create a harmonious flow.

6. REVERSE DIRECTION:

- After completing a set of circles in one direction, reverse the motion.
- This variation targets different muscles in the shoulder and upper back.

7. REPETITIONS:

- Aim for 1-2 minutes of continuous arm circles in each direction.
- Start with smaller circles and gradually progress to larger circles as your muscles warm up.

INSTRUCTIONAL TIPS:

- Maintain a soft bend in your elbows to prevent strain.
- Focus on the quality of the movement rather than speed.
- If you experience any discomfort or fatigue, reduce the size of the circles or take a short break.

Incorporating arm circles into your warm-up routine enhances blood flow, increases joint flexibility, and prepares your upper body for the upcoming Pilates exercises. Remember, smooth and controlled movements contribute to a successful warm-up.

To agile and limber arms.

WALL LEG SWINGS

1. SETTING UP:

- Find a clear wall space to stand facing.
- Place your hands on the wall at shoulder height for support.

2. STARTING POSITION:

- Stand with your feet hip-width apart.
- Engage your core muscles for stability.

3. SWINGING FORWARD:

- Lift your right leg forward, keeping it straight.
- Swing your leg gently back and forth in a controlled manner.

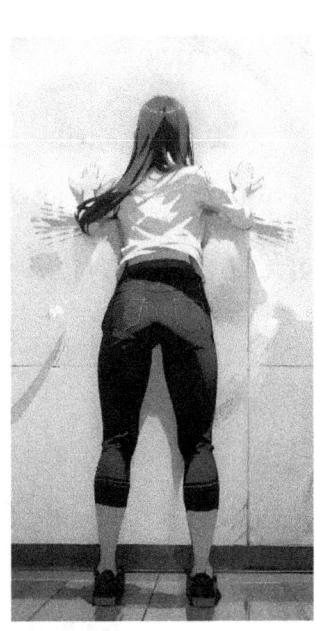

4. SIDE-TO-SIDE SWINGS:

- After completing forward swings, switch to swinging your leg from side to side.
- Maintain control and focus on the movement coming from your hip joint.

5. FOCUS ON FORM:

- Keep your torso stable and avoid excessive leaning.
- Maintain a slight bend in the standing leg for balance.
- Engage your core throughout the swings.

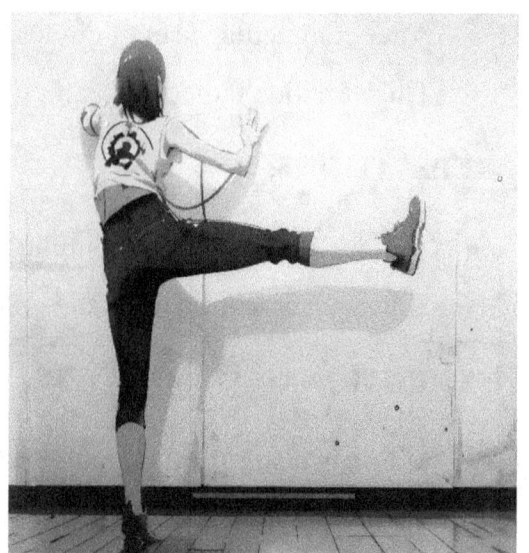

6. BREATHING RHYTHM:

- Inhale as your leg swings forward, and exhale as it swings backward.
- Sync your breath with the rhythmic leg movements.

7. SWITCH LEGS:

Repeat the swings with your left leg, following the same forward and side-to-side sequence.

8. REPETITIONS:

Aim for 15-20 swings with each leg, gradually increasing the range of motion as your muscles warm up.

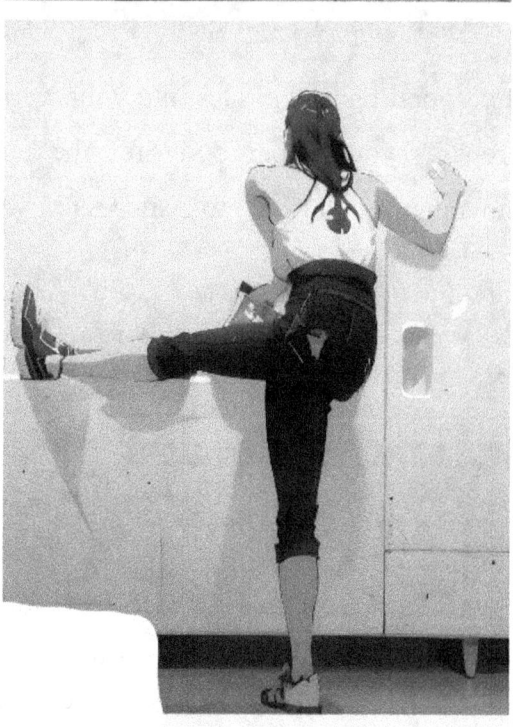

INSTRUCTIONAL TIPS:

- Start with smaller swings and gradually increase the amplitude as your muscles become more flexible.
- Maintain a relaxed and controlled pace to avoid straining the muscles.
- If you experience discomfort, reduce the range of motion or stop the swings.

Incorporating wall leg swings into your warm-up routine enhances hip mobility and flexibility, preparing your lower body for the demands of Pilates exercises. Remember, controlled and deliberate movements contribute to a safe and effective warm-up.

To limber and agile legs.

WALL ROLL DOWN

1. STARTING POSITION:

- Stand with your back against the wall, ensuring your feet are hip-width apart.
- Keep a slight bend in your knees to avoid locking them.

2. INITIATE THE MOVEMENT:

- Inhale deeply through your nose, engaging your core muscles.
- As you exhale, begin to articulate your spine by tucking your chin towards your chest.

3. SEQUENTIAL MOVEMENT:

- Slowly roll down through each vertebra, aiming to touch the wall one vertebra at a time.
- Allow your arms to hang naturally towards the ground.

4. FORWARD FOLD:

Continue rolling down until your hands reach the floor, or as close as your flexibility allows. Keep a soft bend in your knees throughout the movement.

5. HOLDING THE STRETCH:

Once in the forward fold position, take a moment to feel the stretch along your spine and hamstrings. Breathe deeply, allowing your body to relax into the stretch.

6. RETURNING TO START:

Inhale deeply again and start the ascent by stacking each vertebra back up against the wall.

Ensure a controlled and sequential movement.

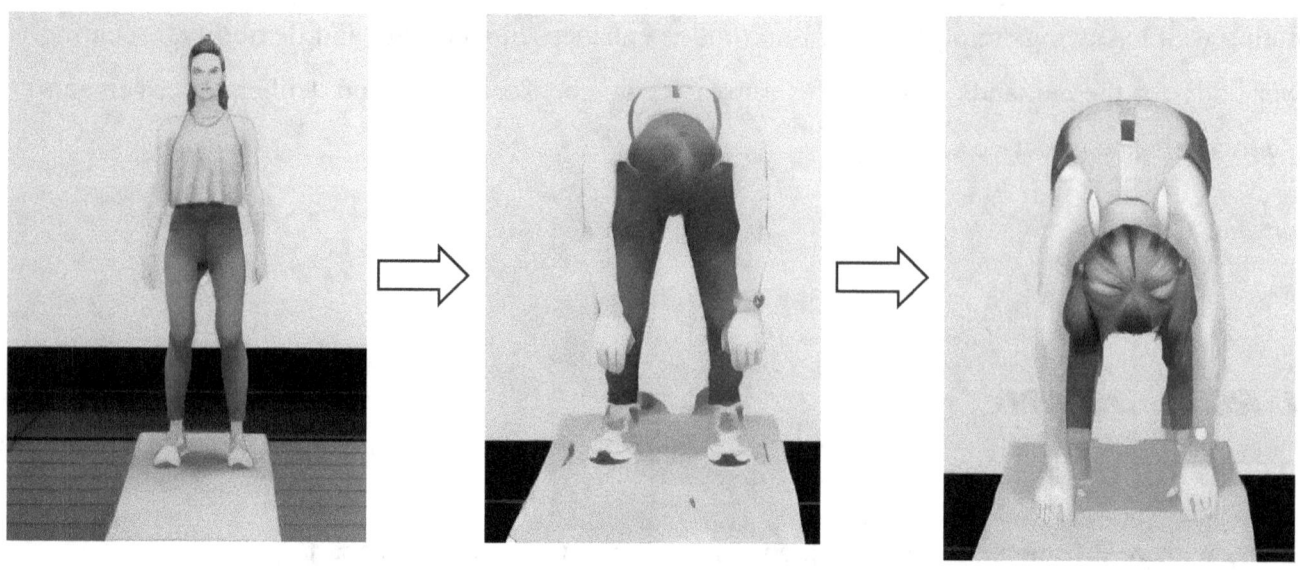

7. FINAL POSITION:

Return to the starting position with your spine against the wall and your body upright.

INSTRUCTIONAL TIPS:

- Maintain a slow and controlled pace throughout the movement.
- Focus on the articulation of each vertebra, creating a smooth and flowing motion.
- Only go as far into the forward fold as your flexibility allows without strain.
- Keep your core engaged to support your spine.

The wall roll-down is an excellent way to release tension in the spine, improve flexibility, and increase body awareness. Incorporate this exercise into your routine to enhance your Pilates practice and overall well-being.

To a supple and agile spine.

SHOULDER ROLLS

1. STARTING POSITION:

- Stand with your feet shoulder-width apart.
- Let your arms hang naturally by your sides.

2. FORWARD SHOULDER ROLLS:

- Begin by lifting your shoulders towards your ears in a circular motion.
- Roll your shoulders forward, moving them in a circular path.
- Continue the forward motion for 10-15 seconds.

3. UPWARD MOVEMENT:

- Transition from the forward roll to lifting your shoulders straight up towards your ears.
- Hold this elevated position for a moment, feeling the stretch in your neck and upper back.

4. REVERSE SHOULDER ROLLS:

- Gradually roll your shoulders backward in a circular motion.
- Feel the tension release as you complete the backward roll.
- Continue the backward motion for 10-15 seconds.

5. DOWNWARD MOVEMENT:

- Transition from the backward roll to lowering your shoulders back to the starting position.
- Allow your shoulders to relax completely before starting the next cycle.

6. REPETITIONS:

Aim for 2-3 sets of 10-15 seconds each for both forward and backward shoulder rolls.

INSTRUCTIONAL TIPS:

- Keep your movements slow and controlled to maximize the stretch.
- Focus on relaxing your neck and upper back during the exercise.
- Breathe naturally and avoid holding your breath.

Shoulder rolls are an excellent way to release tension and increase mobility in the shoulder joints. Incorporate these rolls into your warm-up routine to prepare your upper body for a productive Wall Pilates session.

To relaxed and flexible shoulders. 💀 🧘

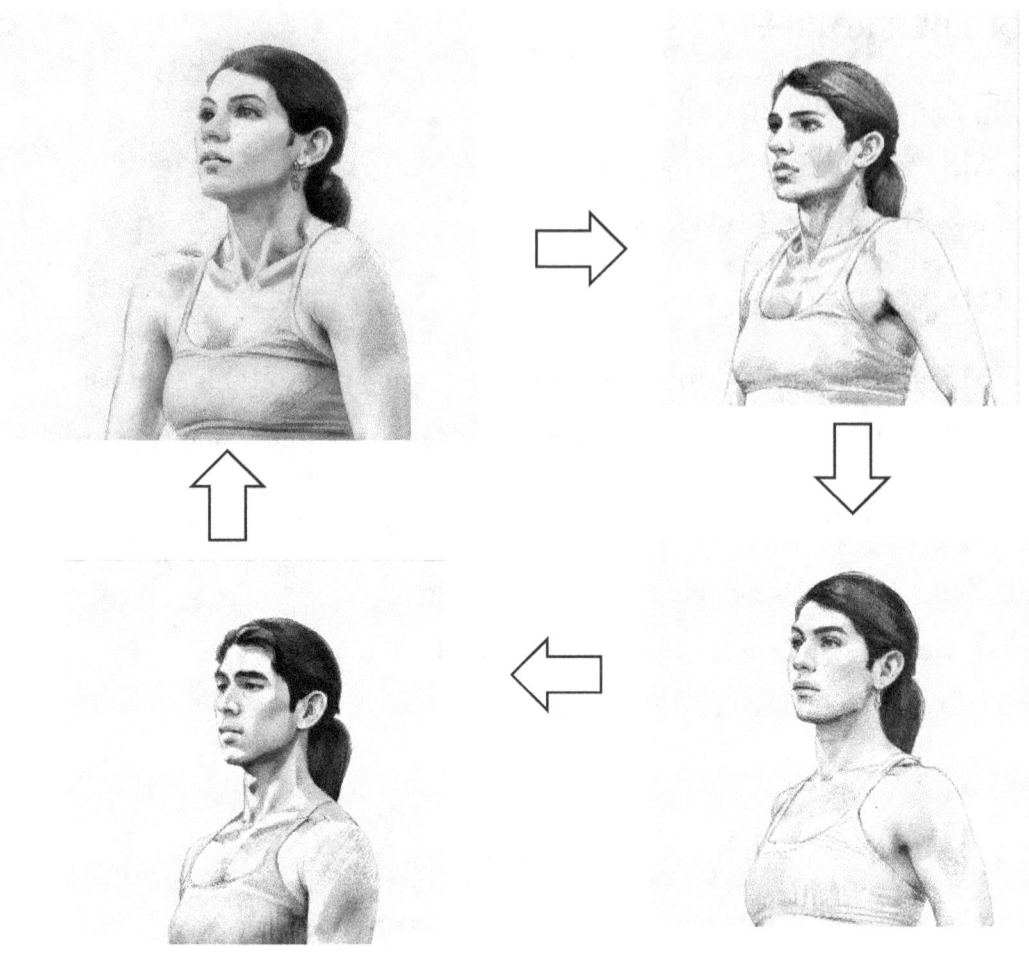

SHOULDER ROLLS

WALL HIP CIRCLES

1. STARTING POSITION:

- Stand facing the wall, with your feet hip-width apart.
- Place your hands on the wall at chest height for support.

2. CIRCULAR MOTION FORWARD:

- Begin by lifting your right knee towards your chest in a controlled manner.
- Move your right knee out to the side, creating a circular motion.
- Extend your right leg back, completing the circle.
- Repeat the circular motion with your right leg for 30 seconds.

3. SWITCH TO THE LEFT LEG:

- Lower your right leg and repeat the circular motion with your left leg.

- Lift the left knee, move it out to the side, and extend it back in a circular motion.

- Repeat the circular motion with your left leg for 30 seconds.

4. FOCUS ON FORM:

- Keep your movements controlled and deliberate.

- Engage your core for stability and balance. Maintain a straight spine throughout the exercise.

5. BREATHING RHYTHM:

- Inhale as you lift your knee, and exhale as you extend your leg back.

- Sync your breath with the circular motion to create a smooth flow.

6. REVERSE DIRECTION:

- After completing circles in one direction, reverse the motion.

- Lift your knee, move it to the side, and then forward in a reverse circular motion.

7. REPETITIONS:

- Aim for 30 seconds of continuous hip circles in each direction for both legs.

- Gradually increase the duration as your hip mobility improves.

INSTRUCTIONAL TIPS:

- Use the wall for support to maintain balance.

- Focus on the range of motion that feels comfortable for your hips.

- If you experience any discomfort, reduce the size of the circles or perform the exercise with smaller movements.

Incorporating wall hip circles into your warm-up routine enhances flexibility, reduces stiffness, and prepares your hips for the Pilates exercises ahead. Remember, smooth and controlled movements contribute to a successful warm-up.

To fluid and flexible hips.

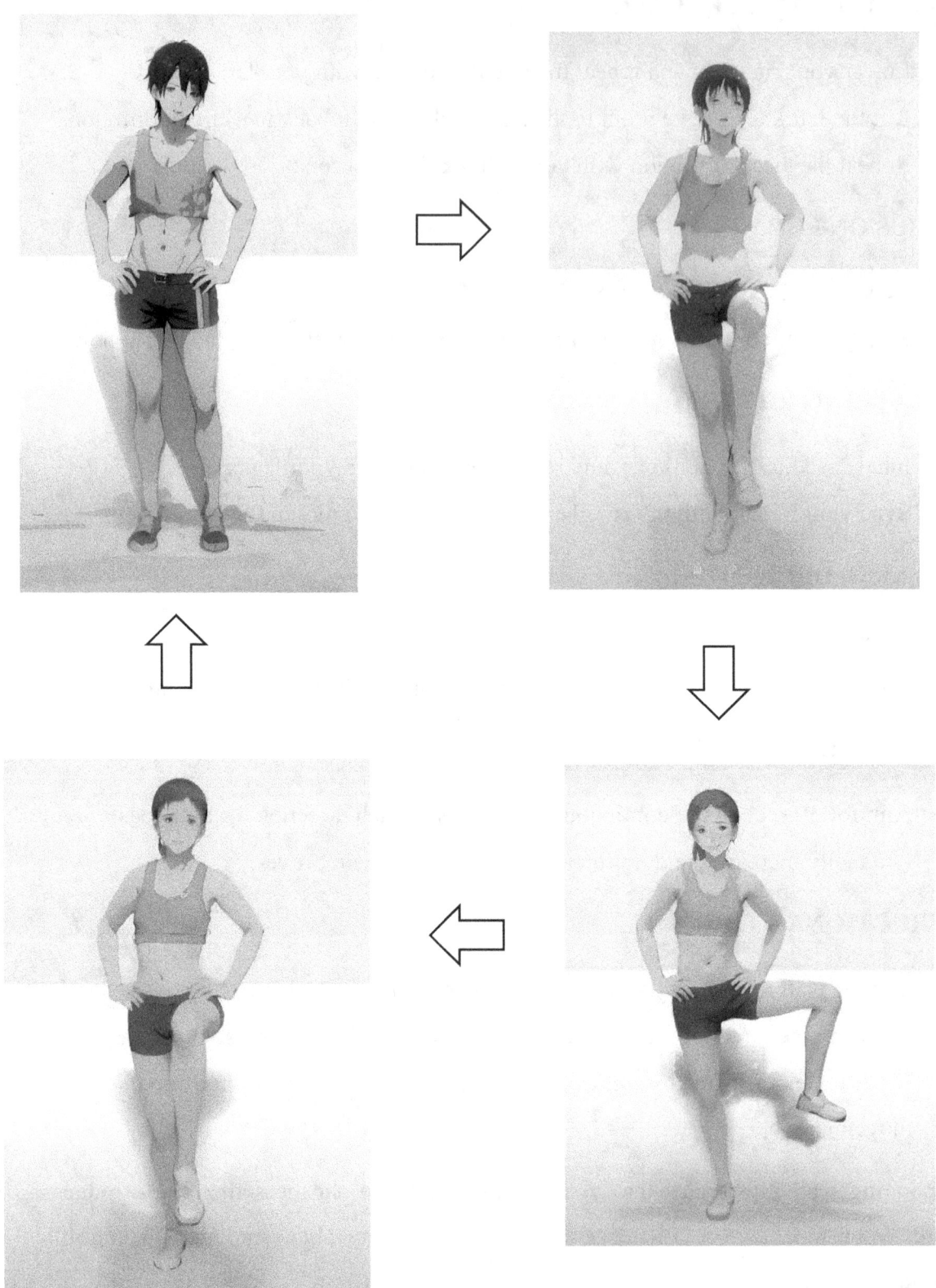

WALL SQUATS

1. STARTING POSITION:

- Stand with your back against a flat wall, ensuring your feet are hip-width apart.
- Keep your feet a few inches away from the wall. Engage your core muscles for stability.

2. LOWERING INTO THE SQUAT:

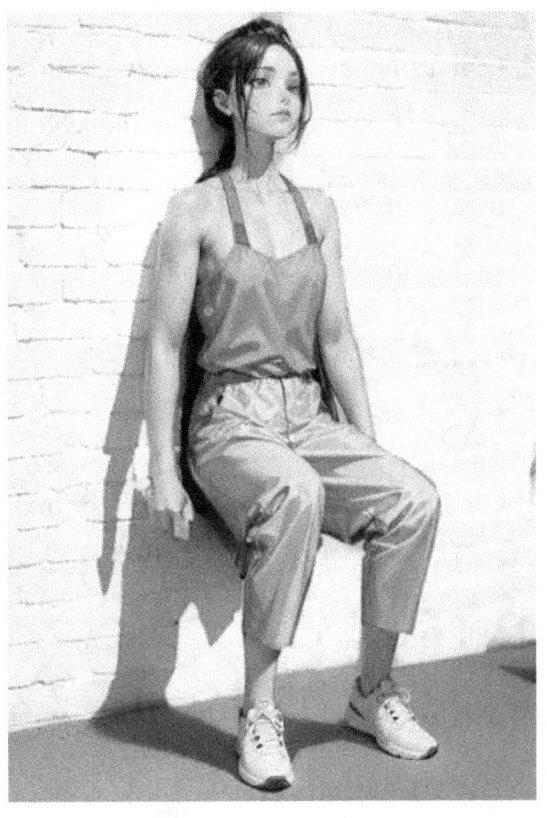

- Slowly slide down the wall, bending your knees and lowering your body into a squat position.
- Aim to lower yourself until your thighs are parallel to the ground or as far as your flexibility allows.

3. KNEE ALIGNMENT:

- Ensure your knees are directly above your ankles, not extending beyond your toes.
- Maintain a neutral spine by keeping your back against the wall.

4. HOLDING THE SQUAT:

- Hold the squat position for 15-30 seconds initially, gradually increasing the duration as your strength improves.
- Focus on distributing your weight evenly between both feet.

5. BREATHING RHYTHM:

- Inhale as you lower into the squat position and exhale as you hold the squat.

6. RISING FROM THE SQUAT:

- Press through your heels to push yourself back up to the starting position.
- Keep the movement controlled and avoid locking your knees at the top.

7. REPETITIONS:

Perform 10-15 repetitions of wall squats, gradually increasing the number as your strength progresses.

INSTRUCTIONAL TIPS:

- Maintain a slow and controlled pace throughout the exercise.
- Focus on the engagement of your quadriceps, hamstrings, and glutes.
- If you experience any discomfort or strain, adjust the depth of your squat or consult with a fitness professional.

Wall squats are an excellent way to build lower body strength and endurance. Incorporate them into your Wall Pilates routine to sculpt and tone your legs while improving overall stability.

To strong and toned legs.

ANKLE CIRCLES

1. STARTING POSITION:

- Sit comfortably on the floor or on a mat.
- Extend your legs straight in front of you.

2. LIFT ONE LEG:

Lift one foot off the ground, keeping the other leg extended.

3. CIRCULAR MOTION:

- Begin by rotating your ankle in a circular motion.
- Start with clockwise circles and then switch to counterclockwise.

4. VARY THE SIZE:

- Initiate with small circles and gradually increase the size as your ankle warms up.
- Focus on maintaining control and precision in the movement.

5. SWITCH LEGS:

- After completing circles with one ankle, switch to the other leg.
- Repeat the circular motion in both directions.

6. FLEX AND POINT:

- While the foot is lifted, alternate between pointing your toes and flexing your foot.
- This additional movement enhances ankle flexibility.

7. REPETITIONS:

- Aim for 1-2 minutes of ankle circles on each leg.
- Perform a sufficient number of rotations to ensure the ankles are adequately warmed up.

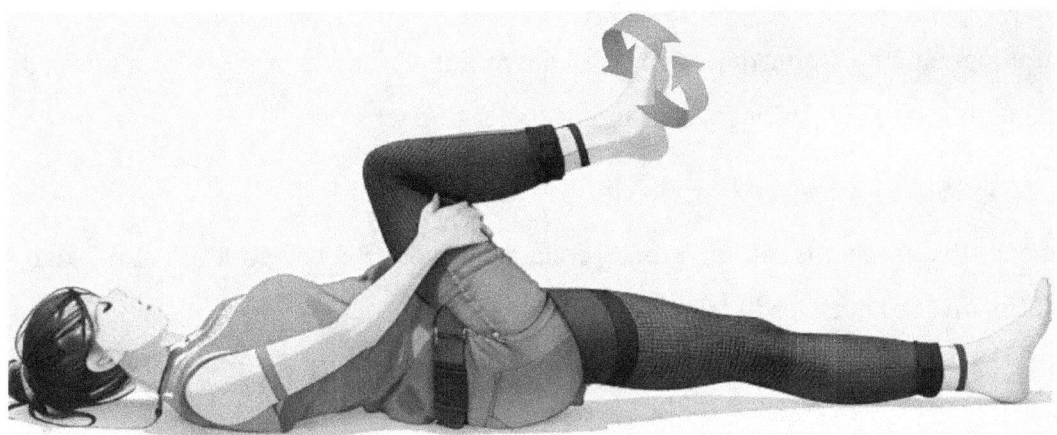

INSTRUCTIONAL TIPS:

Keep the movement controlled and deliberate to avoid unnecessary strain.

Maintain a straight posture with a slight lean back using your hands for support.

Breathe rhythmically throughout the exercise to enhance relaxation.

Adding ankle circles to your warm-up routine improves ankle mobility, crucial for a variety of Pilates exercises. Remember, this simple yet effective movement contributes to a smoother and more comfortable workout experience.

To nimble and agile ankles.

COOLING DOWN: THE ESSENTIAL WIND-DOWN

The cooling down phase is a crucial component of your Pilates routine, providing a gentle transition from the intensity of the workout to a state of relaxation. Follow this step-by-step guide to perform the essential wind-down effectively.

1. GENTLE MOVEMENT:

Start by incorporating slow and controlled movements that mimic the exercises you performed during the session. This helps gradually lower your heart rate and ease your body into a more relaxed state.

2. DEEP BREATHING:

Emphasize deep diaphragmatic breathing during the cool down. Inhale slowly through your nose, allowing your abdomen to expand, and exhale through your mouth, releasing tension.

3. STATIC STRETCHES:

Focus on static stretches that target the muscle groups engaged in your Pilates workout. Hold each stretch for 15-30 seconds, allowing the muscles to lengthen and relax.

4. NECK STRETCHES:

Gently tilt your head from side to side, forward and backward, to release tension in the neck and shoulders. Perform slow and controlled movements, avoiding any sudden jerks.

5. SHOULDER ROLLS:

Roll your shoulders in a circular motion, both forward and backward. This helps alleviate shoulder tightness and enhances overall upper body flexibility.

6. SPINE STRETCHES:

Incorporate stretches that focus on the spine, such as seated twists or gentle spinal rotations. Move within your comfortable range of motion, allowing the spine to decompress.

7. FULL-BODY AWARENESS:

Consciously relax each part of your body, starting from your toes and working your way up to your head. Bring awareness to any areas of residual tension and release it through intentional relaxation.

8. MINDFULNESS AND GRATITUDE:

Take a few moments to center your mind and express gratitude for the effort you put into your Pilates practice. Connect with a sense of accomplishment and well-being.

9. HYDRATION:

Rehydrate by drinking water to replenish fluids lost during the workout. Proper hydration supports muscle recovery and overall well-being.

10. REFLECTION:

Reflect on the positive aspects of your workout, acknowledging any progress or achievements. Use this time for mental and emotional rejuvenation. Incorporating a thorough cool down into your Pilates routine is essential for promoting flexibility, preventing muscle stiffness, and fostering a sense of calmness.

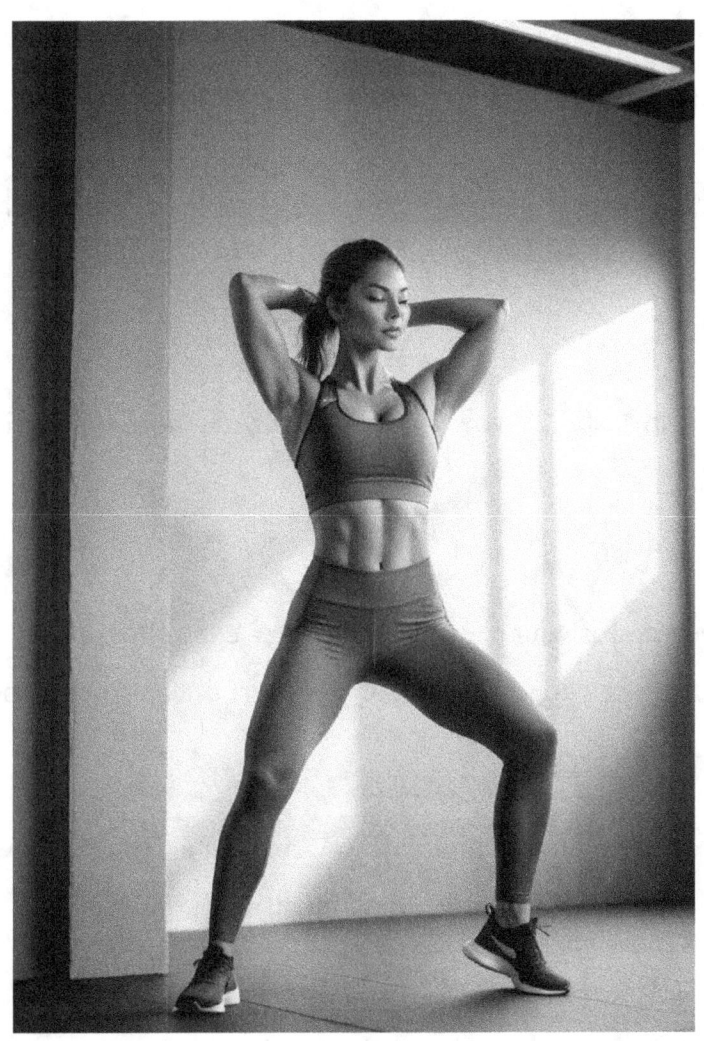

CHAPTER 5 - CORE EXERCISES: SCULPT & STRENGTHEN YOUR CORE.

Welcome to the heart of your wall Pilates journey—core exercises that will not only sculpt your midsection but also enhance your overall strength and stability. Follow this guide to engage and strengthen your core muscles effectively.

WALL MOUNTAIN CLIMBERS

Wall mountain climbers are dynamic and effective exercises that engage multiple muscle groups, primarily targeting the core, shoulders, and legs. Follow this step-by-step guide to perform wall mountain climbers with proper form and maximize their benefits.

STARTING POSITION:

- Begin in a high plank position facing the wall, with your hands placed shoulder-width apart on the wall.
- Ensure your wrists are aligned with your shoulders, and your body forms a straight line from head to heels.

ENGAGE YOUR CORE:

Tighten your abdominal muscles to stabilize your spine. Keep your hips level with your shoulders throughout the exercise.

BRING KNEES TO CHEST:

- Alternately bring one knee towards your chest, maintaining a controlled and deliberate movement.
- Use your core muscles to draw the knee as close to your chest as comfortably possible.

FOCUS ON RHYTHMIC MOVEMENT:

- Execute the exercise in a smooth and rhythmic fashion, creating a dynamic flow.
- Maintain a steady pace to elevate your heart rate and intensify the workout.

ALTERNATE LEG MOVEMENT:

As one knee returns to the starting position, swiftly bring the other knee towards your chest. Continue to alternate between legs, mimicking a climbing motion against the wall.

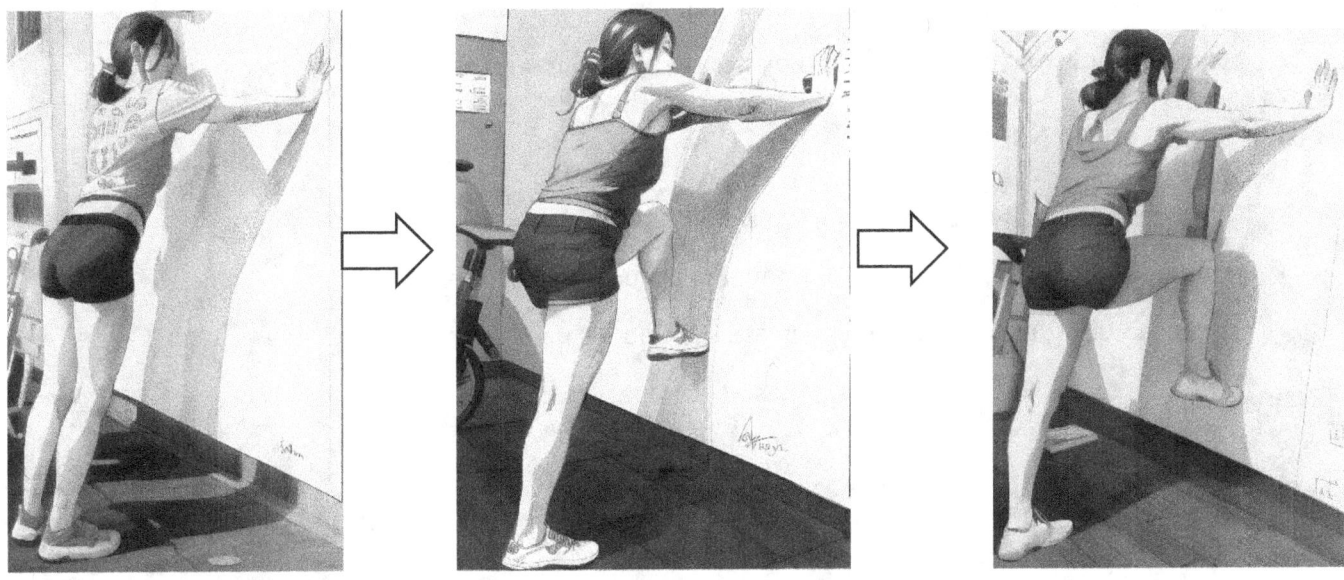

WATCH YOUR FORM:

Pay attention to your form throughout the exercise to prevent sagging or arching in the lower back. Keep your shoulders directly over your wrists for optimal stability.

MODIFY AS NEEDED:

If you're a beginner, start with a slower pace and gradually increase the speed as you build strength. Feel free to modify the exercise by bringing your knees towards your chest at a comfortable range.

COMPLETE THE SET:

Perform the wall mountain climbers for the desired duration or as part of a structured workout routine. Aim for consistency in your movements to maximize the effectiveness of the exercise.

Remember to maintain control, focus on your breathing, and listen to your body. Wall mountain climbers can be tailored to various fitness levels.

To a strong and engaged core.

ISOMETRIC WALL PLANK HOLD

1. SETUP:

- Position yourself facing the wall, about arm's length away.
- Place your palms flat against the wall, shoulder-width apart.
- Extend your arms fully, ensuring they are parallel to the ground.

2. BODY ALIGNMENT:

- Maintain a straight line from your head to your heels.
- Engage your core by drawing your navel towards your spine.
- Squeeze your glutes and thighs to create a stable base.

3. HEAD POSITION:

- Keep your head in a neutral position, aligning it with your spine.
- Avoid dropping or lifting your head to maintain proper spinal alignment.

4. GAZE:

- Direct your gaze towards the wall to maintain a neutral neck position.
- Focus on a point slightly below eye level for optimal alignment.

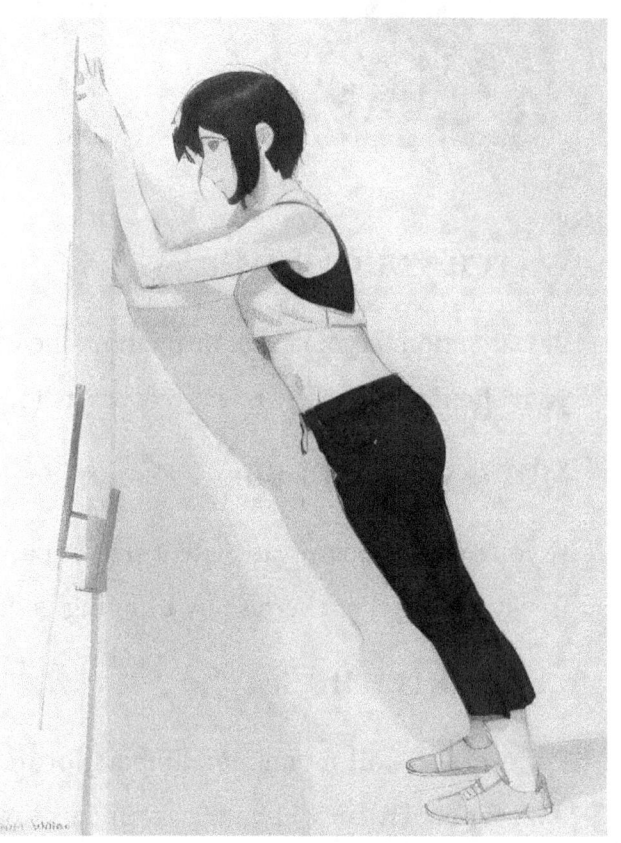

5. HOLDING POSITION:

- Hold the plank position for the desired duration, starting with 15-30 seconds.
- Gradually increase the duration as your strength improves.

6. BREATHING:

Breathe deeply and consistently throughout the hold. Inhale through your nose and exhale through your mouth to stay relaxed.

7. MODIFICATIONS:

If needed, you can perform the isometric wall plank hold with your elbows bent at a 90-degree angle. This modification reduces strain on the shoulders while still engaging the core.

8. COMMON MISTAKES TO AVOID:

Avoid letting your hips sag or pike upward. Keep your body in a straight line. Ensure your shoulders are directly above your wrists to maintain proper alignment.

9. GRADUAL PROGRESSION:

As you build strength, challenge yourself by increasing the duration of the hold. Experiment with different arm positions or leg lifts to add variety and intensity.

10. SAFETY TIPS:

Listen to your body and discontinue the hold if you experience discomfort or strain. If you have any pre-existing shoulder or wrist issues, consult with a fitness professional or healthcare provider for personalized guidance.

To a stable and resilient core.

WALL LEG RAISES

1. SETUP:

- Lie on your back with your hips close to the wall.
- Extend your legs upward, resting them against the wall.
- Place your hands by your sides for stability.

2. STARTING POSITION:

Ensure your lower back is pressed firmly against the floor to activate the core. Your legs should be straight, forming a 90-degree angle with the wall.

3. ENGAGE YOUR CORE:

Inhale deeply, drawing your navel towards your spine. Activate your core muscles to stabilize your pelvis.

4. LOWERING PHASE:

- Exhale as you slowly lower your legs towards the floor.
- Keep the movement controlled, avoiding any sudden or jerky motions.
- Lower your legs only as far as you can while maintaining control and without arching your lower back.

5. LIFTING PHASE:

- Inhale as you raise your legs back up towards the wall.
- Focus on using your lower abdominal muscles to lift your legs.
- Keep the movement smooth and controlled.

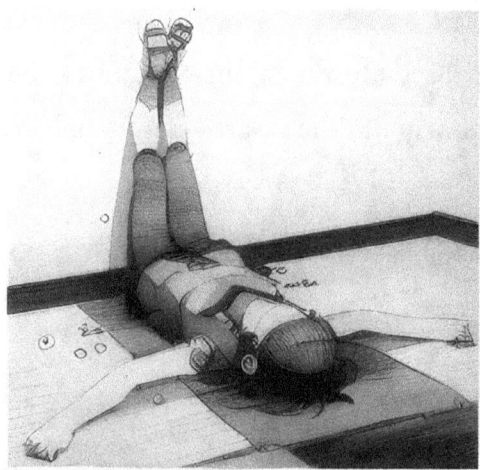 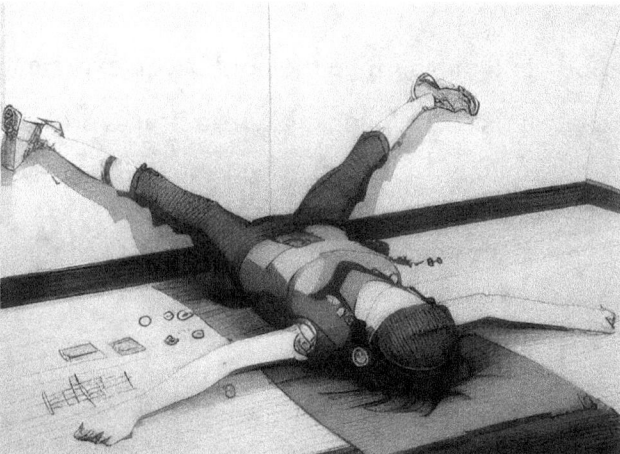

6. REPETITION:

- Perform the exercise for the desired number of repetitions, typically 10-15 repetitions for beginners.
- As you progress, you can gradually increase the number of repetitions.

7. REST AND BREATHING:

Take short breaks between sets to allow your muscles to recover. Breathe consistently throughout the exercise, coordinating your breath with the movement.

8. FORM CHECK:

Regularly check your form to ensure your lower back remains in contact with the floor. If you experience any discomfort in your lower back, modify the range of motion or elevate your legs higher on the wall.

9. VARIATIONS:

Once you've mastered the basic wall leg raises, consider exploring variations to intensify the workout.

Options include adding ankle weights or incorporating a slight pelvic tilt.

10. LISTEN TO YOUR BODY:

Pay attention to how your body responds to the exercise. If you feel any strain or discomfort, modify the movement or consult with a fitness professional.

WALL OBLIQUE CRUNCHES

1. STARTING POSITION:

- Stand with your side facing the wall, about an arm's length away.
- Place your right hand on the wall at shoulder height for support.
- Position your feet hip-width apart and slightly bend your knees.

2. HAND PLACEMENT:

- Extend your left arm overhead, creating a straight line with your body.
- Ensure that your core is engaged, and your spine is in a neutral position.

3. OBLIQUE CRUNCH:

- Initiate the movement by bringing your left knee up towards your left elbow in a controlled manner.
- Simultaneously, perform a side crunch by bringing your left elbow down towards your left knee.
- Focus on contracting your left oblique muscles throughout the movement.

4. EXTENSION:

Return to the starting position by extending your left arm overhead and lowering your left knee.

Maintain a controlled and deliberate pace to maximize muscle engagement.

5. REPEAT ON THE OTHER SIDE:

- After completing the desired number of repetitions on one side, switch to the other side.
- Place your left hand on the wall, extend your right arm overhead, and perform oblique crunches on the opposite side.

TIPS:

Keep your movements controlled to target the oblique muscles effectively. Exhale as you crunch, emphasizing the contraction of the obliques. Focus on quality over quantity, ensuring proper form throughout the exercise.

BENEFITS:

- Targets the oblique muscles, promoting a defined waistline.
- Enhances core strength and stability.
- Improves overall body control and balance.

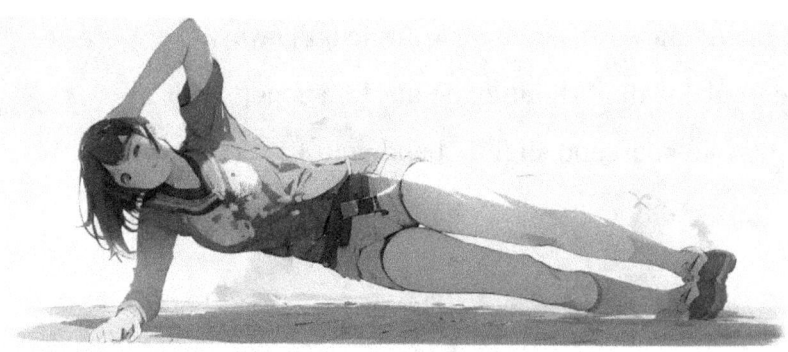

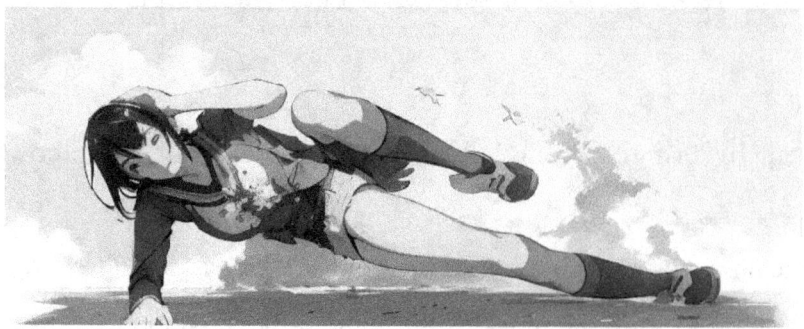

VERTICAL WALL SIT & TWIST

1. STARTING POSITION:

- Stand with your back against the wall, ensuring your feet are hip-width apart.
- Lower your body into a sitting position, sliding down the wall until your knees are bent at a 90-degree angle.

2. CORE ENGAGEMENT:

- Activate your core by pulling your belly button towards your spine.
- Maintain a straight spine and avoid arching your back.

3. HAND PLACEMENT:

- Place your hands together in a prayer position at chest level.
- Keep your elbows out to the sides to allow for a full range of motion.

4. TWISTING MOTION:

While maintaining the wall sit position, twist your torso to one side. Rotate from your waist, bringing your hands towards the wall on the side you are twisting.

5. RETURN TO CENTER:

Slowly return to the center, aligning your hands with your chest.

6. TWIST TO THE OPPOSITE SIDE:

Repeat the twisting motion, this time to the opposite side. Keep the movement controlled and focus on engaging your oblique muscles.

7. REPETITIONS:

Aim for 10-15 repetitions on each side, or as per your fitness level.

TIPS:

- Ensure your knees are directly above your ankles during the wall sit.
- Keep your weight in your heels to activate the muscles in your glutes and thighs.
- Perform the twists in a controlled manner to maximize the engagement of your core muscles.

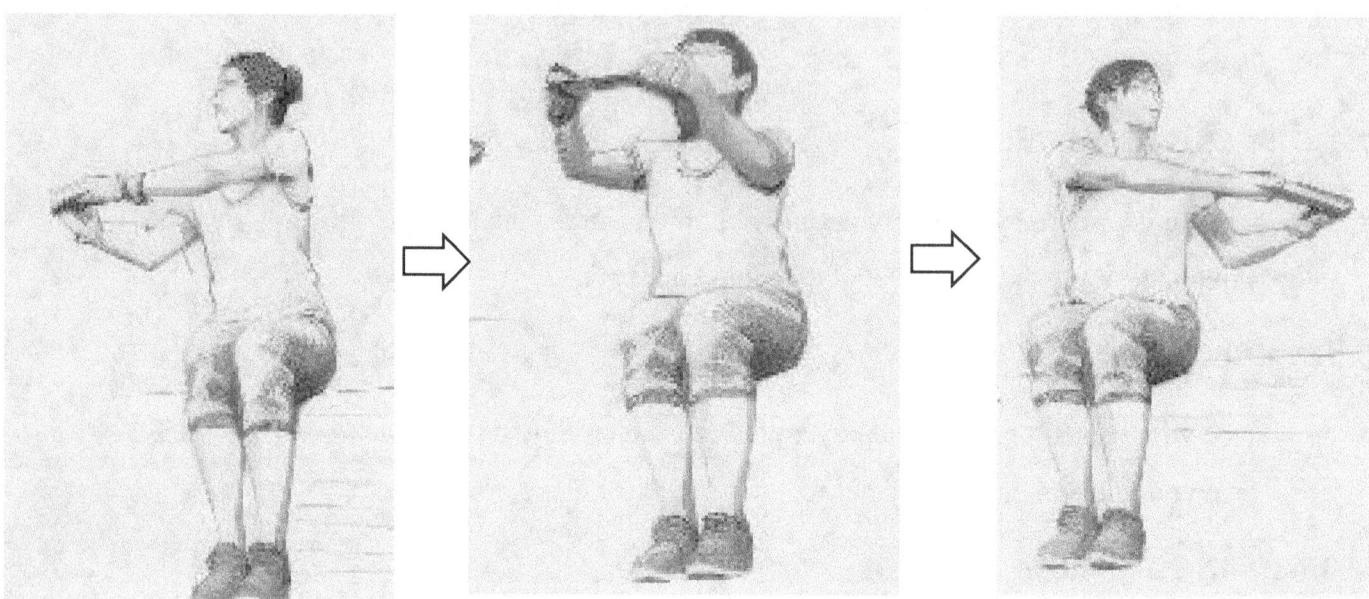

BENEFITS:

The Vertical Wall Sit & Twist not only targets your core but also works on enhancing spinal mobility and improving posture. Regular incorporation of this exercise into your wall Pilates routine will contribute to increased strength, stability, and overall fitness.

WALL DEAD BUG

STARTING POSITION:

- Try to get as much of your spine in contact with the floor by lying flat on your back on a mat or the floor.
- Raise your arms upwards to the ceiling and use your legs to form a "tabletop" by bending your hips and knees to a 90-degree angle.

ENGAGE YOUR CORE:

- Focus on contracting your abdominal muscles to stabilize your spine.
- Maintain contact between your lower back and the floor.
- Raise your left arm over your head and extend your right leg without letting your spine leave the ground.
- As you extend, push your heel aside and bring your toes back towards your body, as though you were standing on that leg.
- When you get to the movement's longest segment, completely exhale.
- Carefully take a step back to the setup position without letting your heel hit the ground.

SWITCH SIDES:

Bring your right arm back to the starting position as you raise your left arm overhead.

At the same time, raise your right leg back to the tabletop position.

CONTINUED ALTERNATION:

Continue alternating arm and leg movements in a controlled and deliberate manner.

Keep the pace steady, emphasizing the engagement of your core.

BREATHING TECHNIQUE:

Coordinate your breath with your movements.

Inhale as you extend your arm and leg, and exhale as you return to the starting position.

REPEAT AND PROGRESS:

Aim for 10 to 15 repetitions on each side, gradually increasing as your strength improves.

Focus on maintaining proper form throughout the exercise.

TIPS:

Avoid arching your lower back by keeping it firmly pressed against the floor.

If you find it challenging, reduce the range of motion until you build sufficient strength.

Pay attention to the connection between your breath and movements for optimal control.

The wall dead bug is an excellent exercise for building core strength and stability. Incorporate it into your wall Pilates routine for a well-rounded and effective workout.

To a strong and stable core

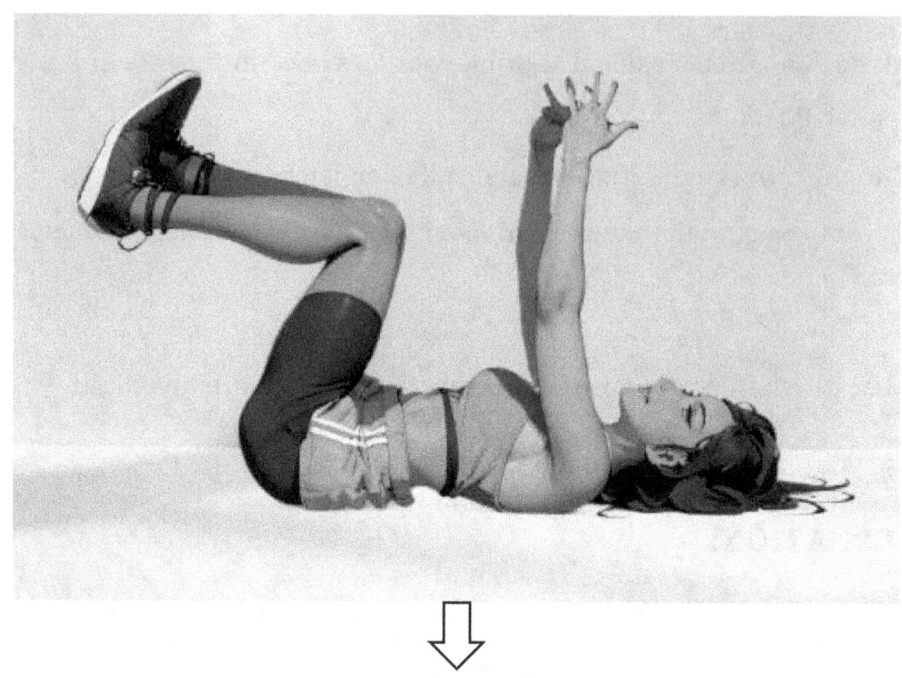

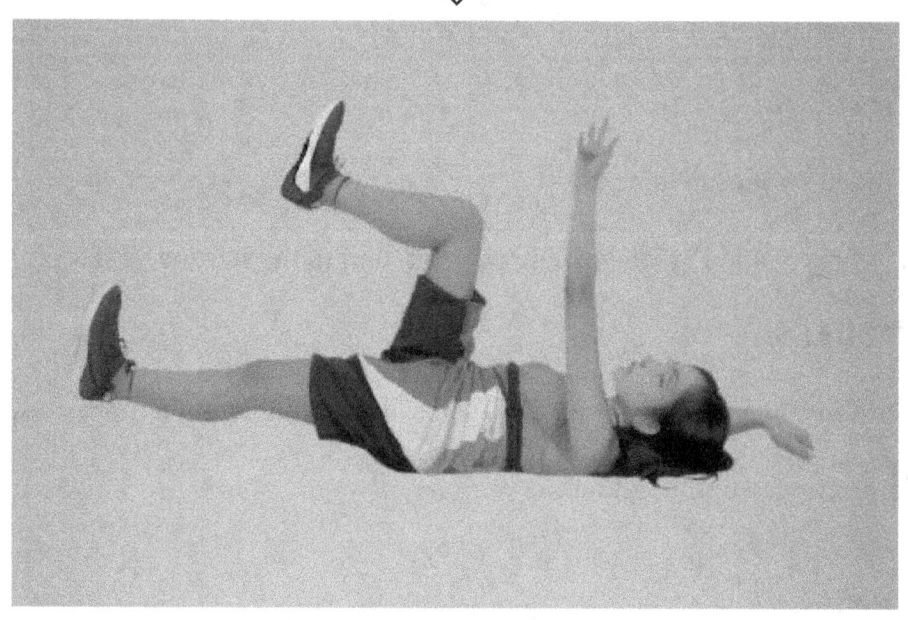

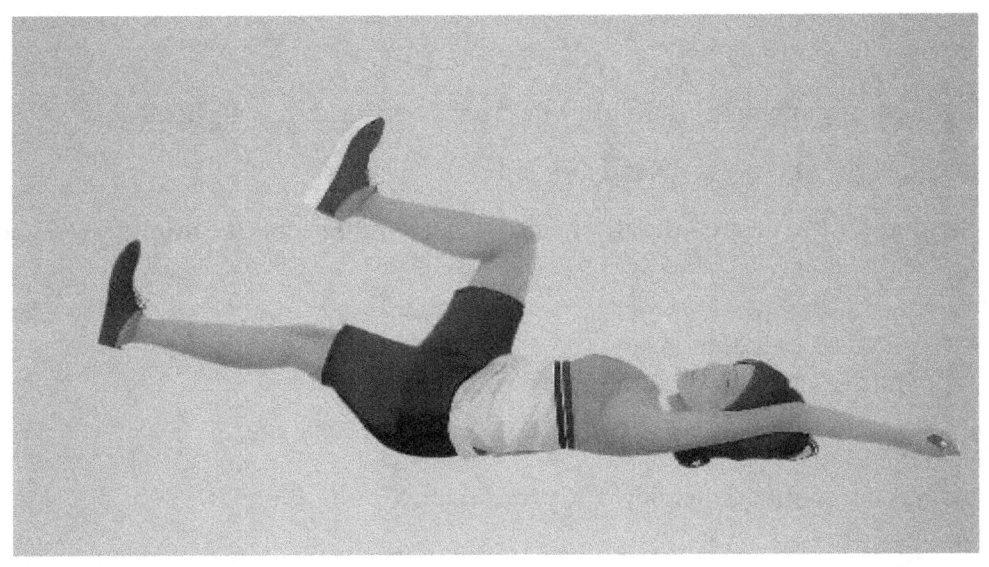

WALL DEAD BUG

WALL SIDE PLANK

STARTING POSITION:

- Stand beside a wall with your feet hip-width apart.
- Place your forearm on the wall, ensuring it's parallel to the ground.
- Keep your elbow directly beneath your shoulder.

ALIGNMENT:

- Stack your feet on top of each other.
- Engage your core muscles to maintain a straight line from your head to your heels.
- Avoid sagging or arching your back.

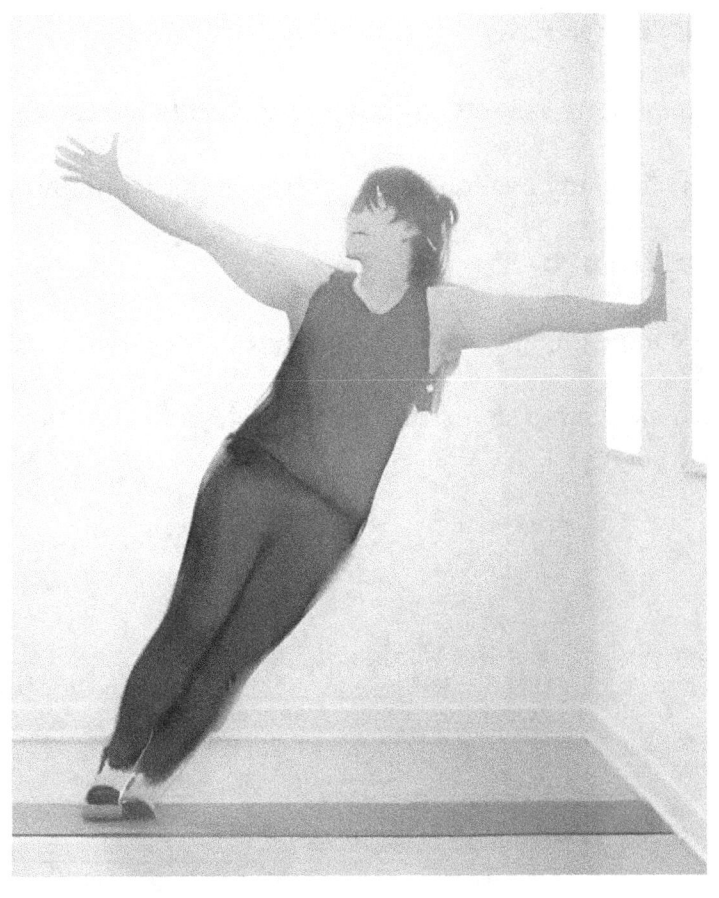

EXECUTION:

- Lift your hips upward, creating a straight line from your head to your heels.
- Focus on keeping your body stable and aligned.
- Hold the position for the desired duration, aiming for 15-30 seconds initially.

BREATHING:

- Breathe deeply and evenly throughout the exercise.
- Inhale through your nose, expanding your ribcage.
- Exhale through your mouth, engaging your core muscles.

MODIFICATION:

If the full side plank is too challenging, you can modify by bending your lower knee and placing it on the ground for additional support. Alternatively, you can perform a side plank against the wall with your knees bent and feet against the wall, creating a diagonal line from your head to your knees.

REPETITION:

Aim to perform 2-3 sets on each side, gradually increasing the duration as you build strength and stability.

Focus on quality over quantity, ensuring proper form throughout the exercise.

COOL DOWN:

After completing the wall side plank, gently release the position and return to a standing position.

Take a moment to stretch any tight muscles and transition into the next exercise or cool-down phase.

HIGH WALL KNEE TUCKS (INVERTED)

STARTING POSITION:

Begin by positioning yourself in a plank position with your legs extended towards the wall.

EXECUTION:

- Engage your core muscles to maintain a straight line from your head to your heels, ensuring your wrists are directly under your shoulders.
- Slowly lift one knee towards your chest while maintaining the plank position, using your abdominal muscles to draw the knee in as close as possible.
- Hold the tucked position for a brief moment, feeling the contraction in your core.
- Return the lifted leg to the starting position, keeping your hips stable and maintaining control throughout the movement.
- Repeat the movement on the opposite side, lifting the other knee towards your chest.
- Continue alternating between legs, focusing on controlled movements and maintaining proper form throughout the exercise.

TIPS:

- Keep your shoulders stable and avoid sinking or arching your back during the movement.
- Maintain a steady breathing pattern, inhaling as you lift the knee and exhaling as you return to the starting position.
- Aim to perform the knee tucks with control and precision, focusing on engaging your core muscles effectively.
- Gradually increase the intensity by speeding up the movement or extending the duration of each repetition as you become more comfortable with the exercise.
- Incorporate wall plank with knee tucks into your Pilates routine to target your core muscles effectively and enhance overall strength and stability.

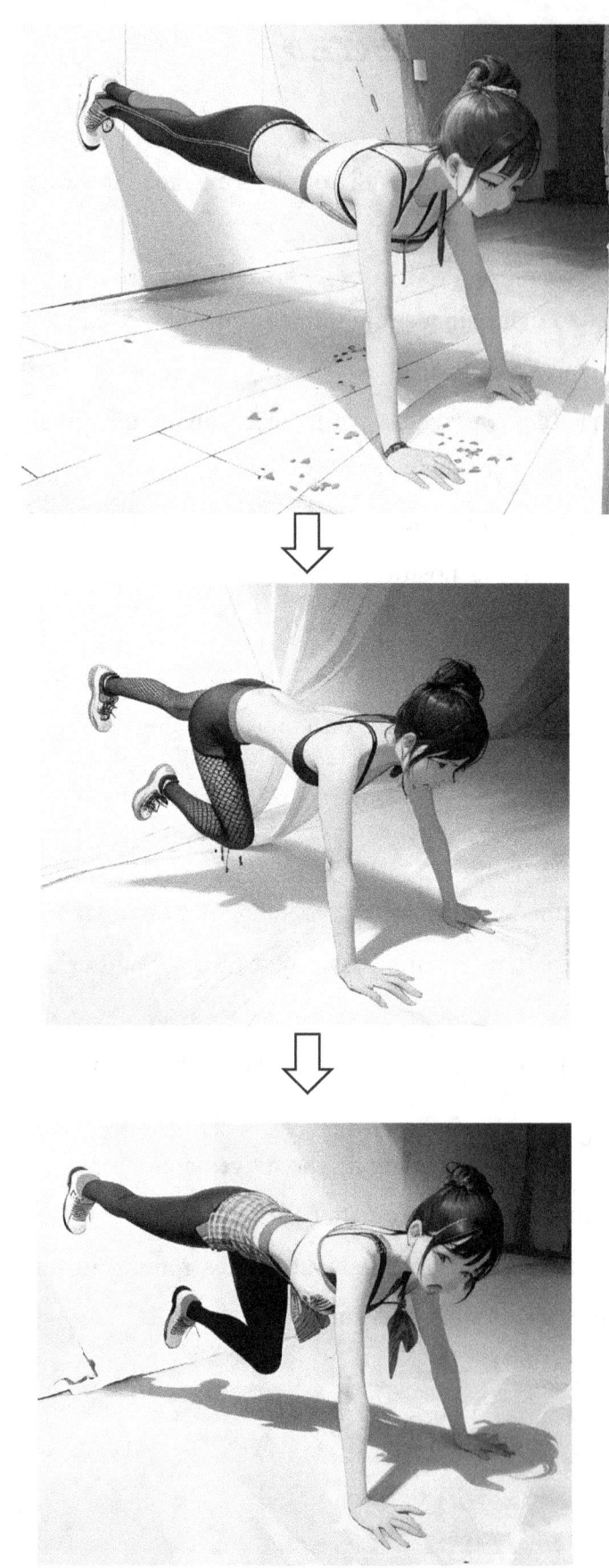

CHAPTER 6 - UPPER BODY EXERCISES: TONE & DEFINE YOUR UPPER BODY

Welcome to the realm of upper body exercises designed to sculpt and define your armsw, shoulders, and upper back. Follow this guide to engage your upper body muscles effectively and achieve that toned and defined look.

WALL ROW

1. STARTING POSITION:

Stand facing the wall with your feet hip-width apart. Extend your arms forward, reaching shoulder height, and imagine grasping handles on the wall.

2. ENGAGE YOUR CORE:

- Tighten your core muscles to stabilize your spine throughout the exercise.
- Maintain a straight posture from your head to your heels.

3. INITIATE THE MOVEMENT:

- Start the movement by pulling your elbows back towards your torso.
- Focus on squeezing your shoulder blades together as you pull.

4. ELBOW POSITION:

- Bend your elbows and aim to bring them close to your sides.
- Keep a controlled and deliberate motion without using momentum.

5. SHOULDER BLADE SQUEEZE:

- At the fully contracted position, emphasize squeezing your shoulder blades together.
- This action engages the muscles in your upper back effectively.

6. CONTROLLED RELEASE:

- Slowly extend your arms back to the starting position, maintaining control over the movement.

- Avoid allowing your shoulders to hunch forward; keep them down and back.

7. REPETITION:

- Perform the wall row for the desired number of repetitions.
- Focus on the quality of each repetition rather than speed.

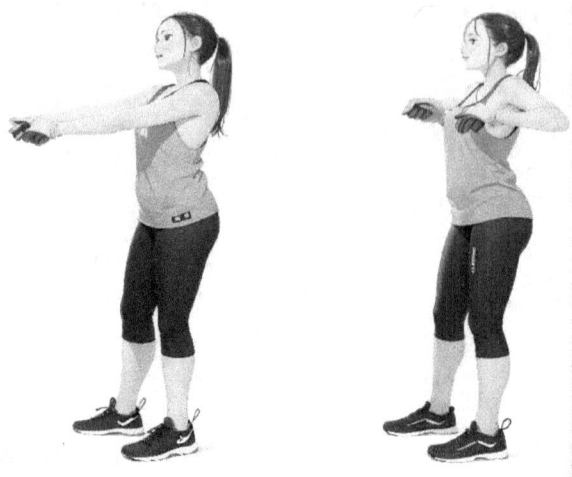

TIPS:

- Breathe naturally throughout the exercise, exhaling as you pull and inhaling during the release.
- Ensure your wrists stay in a neutral position to protect your joints.
- Adjust your distance from the wall to control the exercise intensity.

BENEFITS:

- Strengthens the muscles in the upper back, including the rhomboids and traps.
- Targets the rear deltoids and biceps.
- Improves posture by promoting scapular retraction.

Incorporate wall rows into your upper body workout routine to enhance strength and definition in your back and shoulders.

To a sculpted and toned upper body.

WALL ROW ISOHOLD

1. STARTING POSITION:

- Stand facing the wall with your feet hip-width apart.
- Extend your arms forward, placing your hands on the imaginary handles on the wall.
- Maintain a slight bend in your knees and engage your core for stability.

2. INITIATE THE ROW:

- Pull your elbows back towards your torso, squeezing your shoulder blades together.
- Focus on engaging the muscles in your upper back and avoid using excessive momentum.

3. HOLD THE CONTRACTION:

- Once you've reached the fully contracted position of the row, hold it isometrically.
- Ensure that your shoulder blades are firmly squeezed together, creating tension in your upper back.
- Keep your core engaged and maintain a straight posture throughout the hold.

4. EYE LEVEL ALIGNMENT:

Position your head so that your eyes are level with the imaginary handles on the wall. Avoid tilting your head up or down, maintaining a neutral neck position.

5. BREATHING TECHNIQUE:

Focus on steady and controlled breathing throughout the isohold. Inhale and exhale rhythmically to enhance stability and oxygenation.

6. DURATION:

- Hold the fully contracted position for the desired duration.
- Beginners may start with shorter holds and gradually progress to longer durations as strength improves.

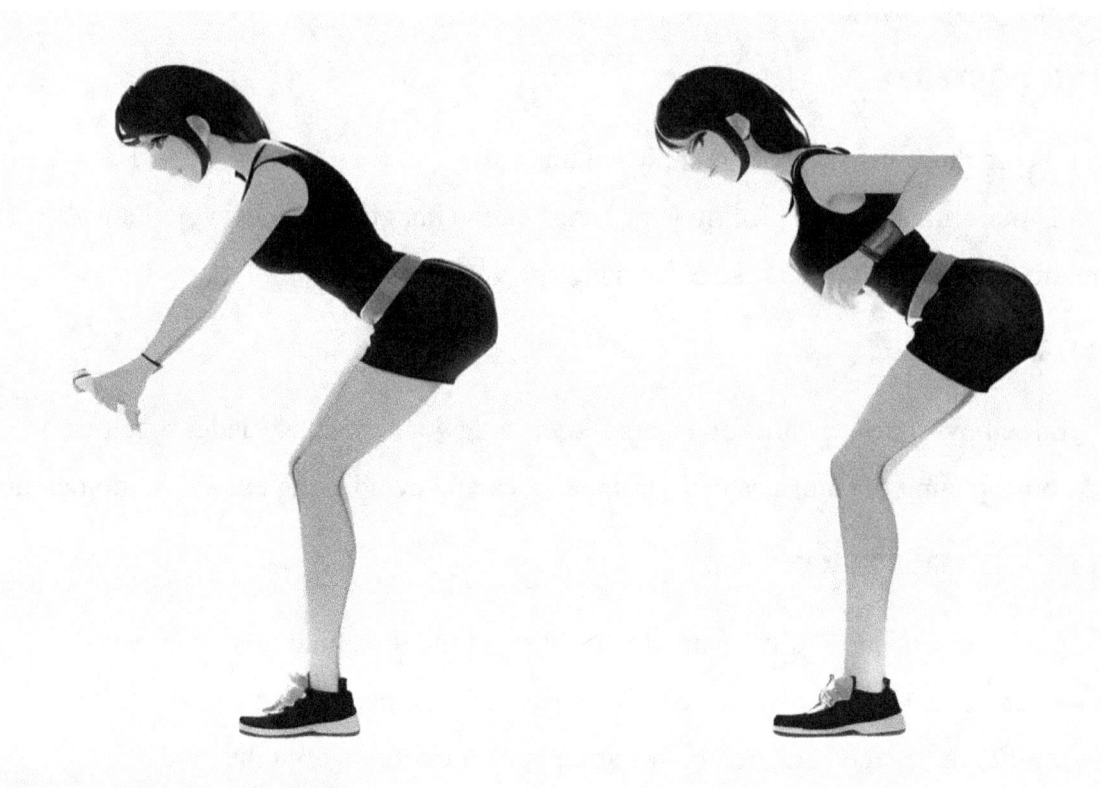

TIPS:

- Keep your shoulders away from your ears, promoting a relaxed neck and shoulder region.
- Maintain a stable lower body by avoiding excessive movement in your hips and knees.
- Visualize squeezing a pencil between your shoulder blades to enhance the engagement of the upper back muscles.

BENEFITS:

- Strengthens the muscles in the upper back, including the rhomboids and trapezius.
- Enhances posture by promoting scapular retraction.
- Targets and tones the shoulders.

HINGE TO WALL

1. STARTING POSITION:

- Stand a few feet away from the wall, facing it.
- Place your feet hip-width apart, ensuring a stable and balanced stance.

2. HAND PLACEMENT:

Extend your arms straight in front of you and place your palms flat against the wall at shoulder height. Your hands should be shoulder-width apart, forming a solid foundation.

3. HIP HINGE:

- Engage your core and hinge at your hips, leaning your upper body forward towards the wall.
- Keep your back straight, maintaining a neutral spine throughout the movement.
- The hinge should primarily come from your hips, allowing your chest to approach the wall.

4. BENDING THE ELBOWS:

- As you hinge forward, bend your elbows to lower your upper body towards the wall.
- Aim to bring your chest close to the wall while keeping your elbows pointing backward.

5. FULL EXTENSION:

- Push through your palms to extend your arms back to the starting position.
- Fully straighten your arms, feeling the contraction in your chest and triceps.

6. REPEAT:

- Perform the hinge to wall exercise for the desired number of repetitions.
- Focus on maintaining proper form and controlled movements throughout.

TIPS:

- Control the movement to maximize engagement in the chest and triceps.
- Keep your core tight to stabilize your spine during the hinge.
- Ensure your wrists, elbows, and shoulders are in alignment for proper joint health.

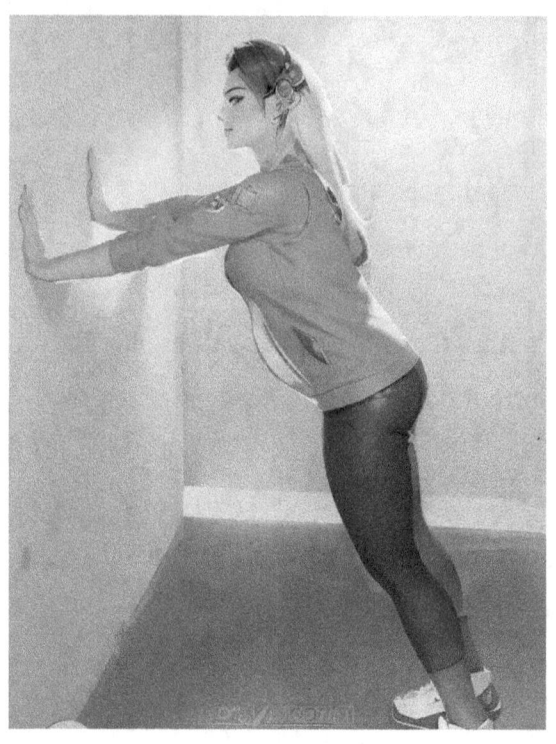 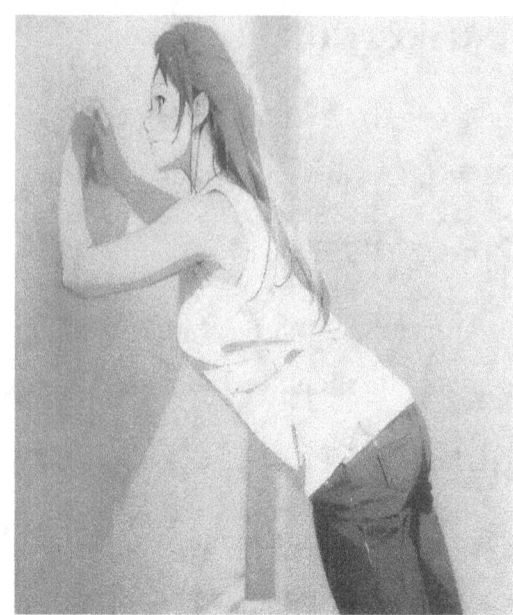

BENEFITS:

- Targets the chest, triceps, and shoulders.
- Enhances upper body strength and endurance.
- Engages the core for stability.

To a sculpted and toned upper body.

WALL TRICEP EXTENSION

1. STARTING POSITION:

- Stand facing the wall with your feet hip-width apart.
- Place your hands on the wall at shoulder height, slightly wider than shoulder-width apart.
- Ensure your body is straight, forming a plank position.

2. LEANING IN:

- Lean your body forward towards the wall, maintaining a straight line from head to heels.
- Keep your elbows close to the wall, pointing backward.

3. BENDING THE ELBOWS:

Lower your body towards the wall by bending your elbows.

Allow your elbows to create a 90-degree angle, bringing your forehead towards the wall.

4. TRICEP CONTRACTION:

Engage your triceps and push through your palms to extend your arms back to the starting position.

Emphasize the contraction in your triceps at the top of the movement.

5. REPETITION:

- Perform the tricep extension for the desired number of repetitions.
- Maintain a controlled pace throughout the exercise to maximize effectiveness.

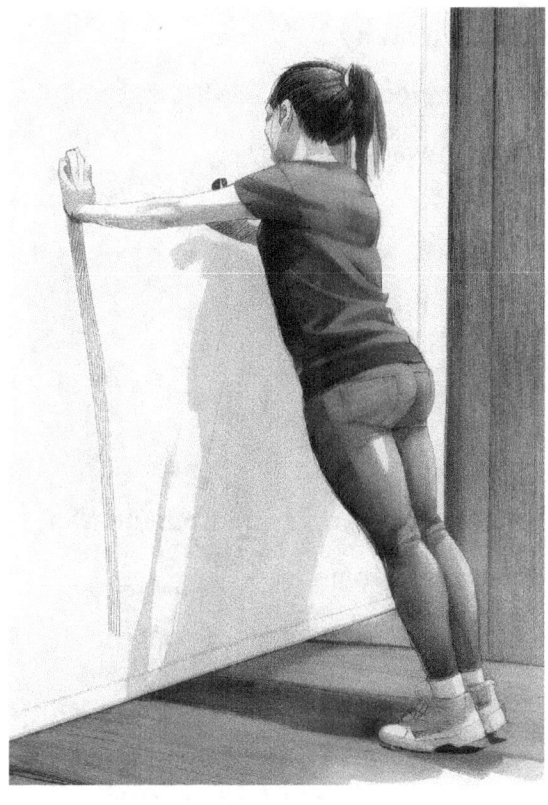 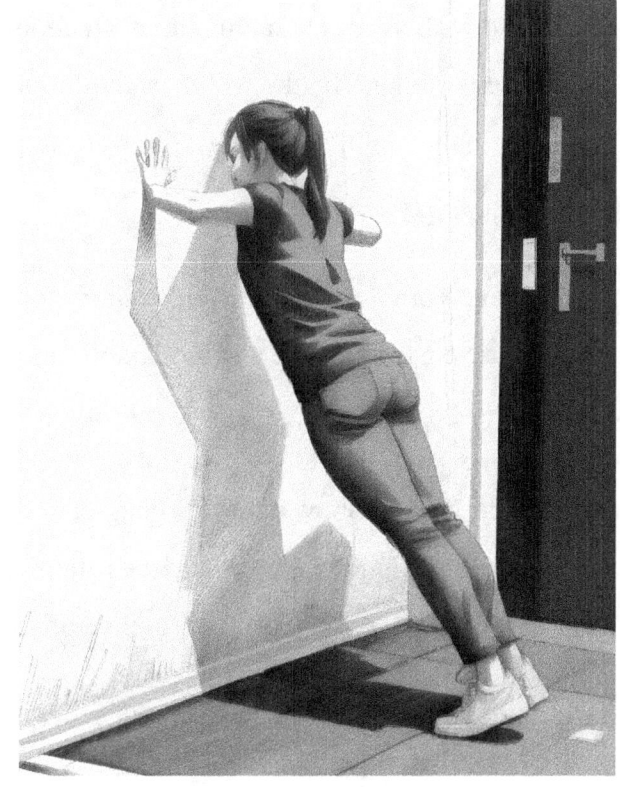

TIPS:

- Focus on keeping your body in a straight line, avoiding any sagging or arching.
- Control the movement to prevent any strain on your shoulders.
- Exhale as you extend your arms and inhale as you bend your elbows.

BENEFITS:

- Targets and tones the triceps, promoting arm strength and definition.
- Engages the core and upper body stabilizing muscles.

Incorporate wall tricep extensions into your upper body routine to enhance arm strength and achieve beautifully toned triceps.

To sculpted arms and strength.

WALL ER (EXTERNAL ROTATION)

1. STARTING POSITION:

- Stand with your side facing the wall, about an arm's length away.
- Place your hand on the wall at shoulder height with your elbow bent at a 90-degree angle.
- Your palm should be against the wall, fingers pointing upward.

2. STABLE CORE:

- Engage your core to maintain stability throughout the exercise.
- Ensure a neutral spine and a relaxed stance.

3. EXTERNAL ROTATION:

- Keeping your elbow bent at 90 degrees, slowly rotate your forearm away from the wall.
- Focus on using the muscles of the rotator cuff to perform the rotation.
- Aim to move only your forearm, keeping the upper arm and shoulder stationary.

4. CONTROLLED MOVEMENT:

- Move in a slow and controlled manner to maximize the effectiveness of the exercise.
- Avoid using momentum or allowing your body to sway.

5. RETURN TO START:

- After reaching the maximum external rotation, slowly bring your forearm back to the starting position.
- Feel the contraction in the muscles of the rotator cuff as you return.

6. REPETITIONS:

- Perform the external rotation for the recommended number of repetitions.
- You can gradually increase resistance by adjusting the distance from the wall or using a resistance band.

TIPS:

- Focus on the quality of the movement rather than speed.
- If you experience any discomfort or pain, stop the exercise and consult with a fitness professional or healthcare provider.

BENEFITS:

- Strengthens the rotator cuff muscles.
- Improves shoulder stability.
- Enhances functional movement patterns.

Incorporate Wall ER into your upper body workout routine to promote shoulder health and build strength in the external rotation muscles.

To strong and resilient shoulders.

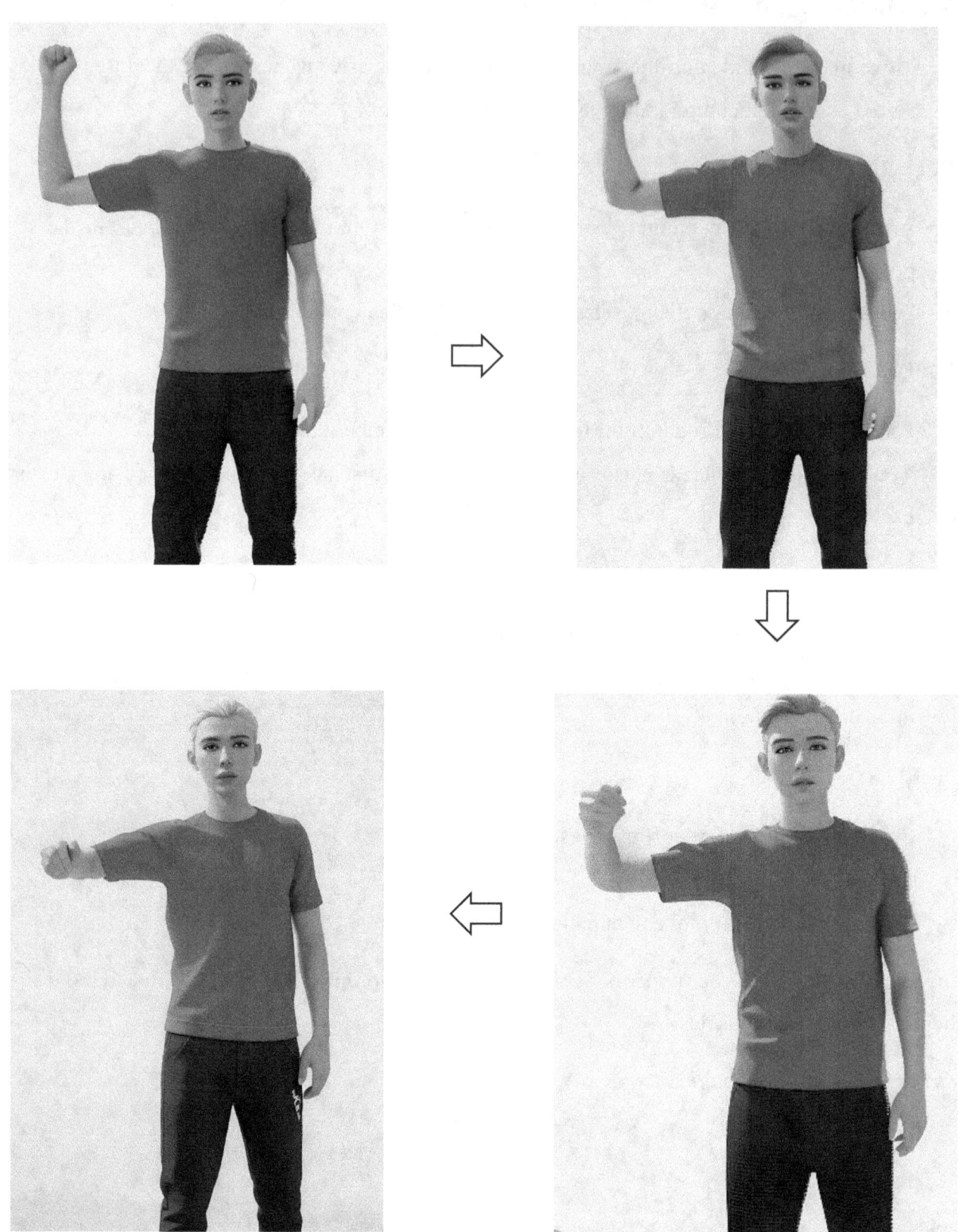

WALL PUSH UP PLUS

1. STARTING POSITION:

- Stand facing the wall with your feet hip-width apart.
- Place your hands on the wall, slightly wider than shoulder-width apart.
- Ensure your body forms a straight line from your head to your heels.

2. PUSH-UP MOTION:

- Lower your chest towards the wall by bending your elbows.
- Keep your core engaged and maintain a straight line from head to heels.
- Lower until your chest is close to the wall, feeling a stretch in your chest and shoulders.

3. PUSH-UP PLUS:

- After completing the standard push-up motion, push through your palms to extend your arms fully.
- This additional movement involves protracting your shoulder blades forward.
- Feel the contraction in your chest and shoulders as you push away from the wall.

4. SHOULDER RETRACTION:

- After the push-up plus, retract your shoulder blades by squeezing them together.
- Emphasize the contraction in your upper back during this phase.
- Your body should return to the starting position with your arms extended.

5. REPETITION:

- Perform the wall push-up plus for the desired number of repetitions.
- Focus on a controlled and deliberate movement to maximize the engagement of your chest and shoulders.

TIPS:

- Keep your body in a straight line throughout the exercise to target the intended muscles effectively.
- Engage your core to maintain stability during the push-up and push-up plus phases.
- Control the descent and ascent to ensure proper muscle engagement.

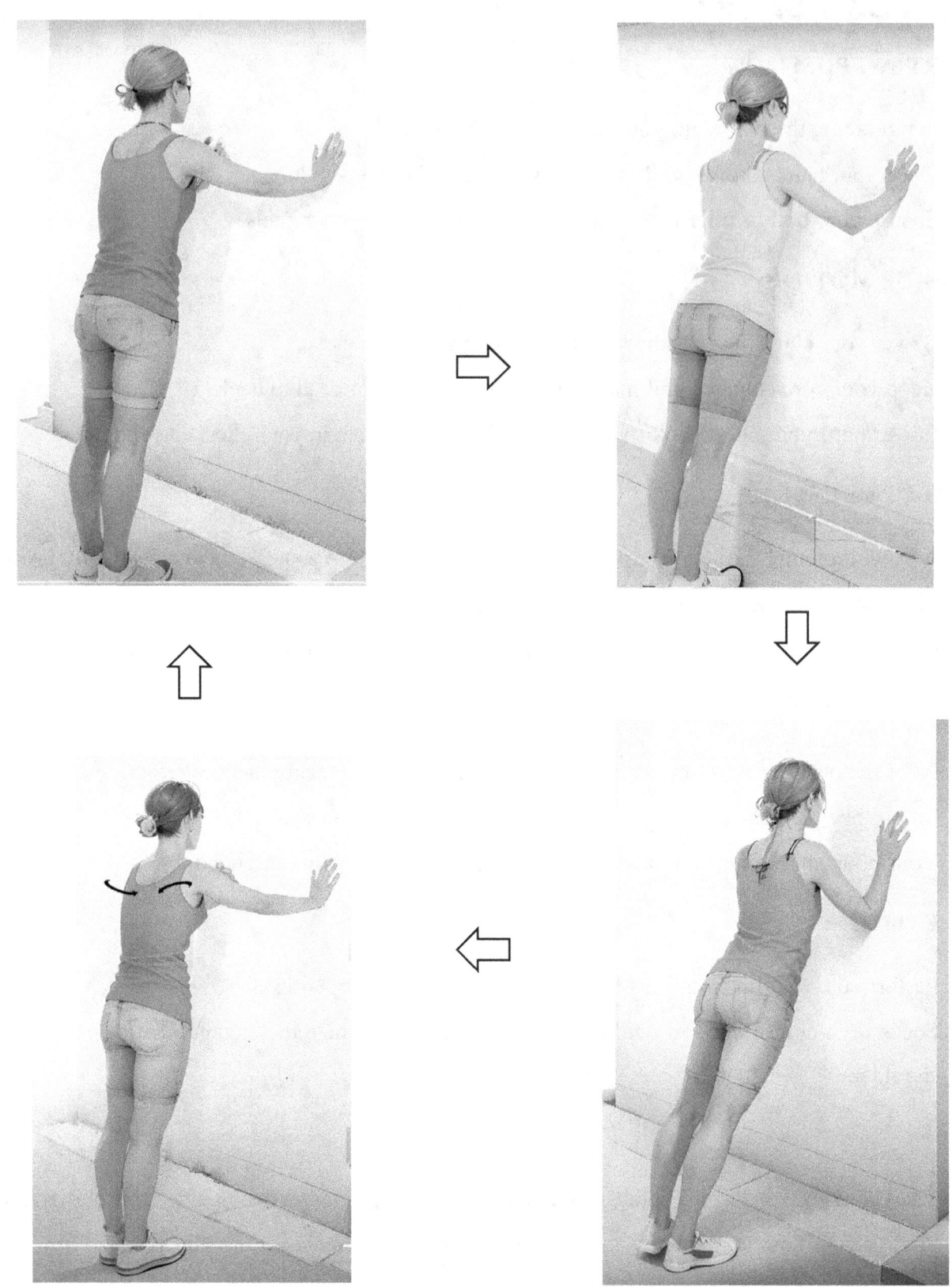

BENEFITS:

- Targets the chest, shoulders, and triceps.

- Enhances shoulder stability and scapular movement.

- Provides a dynamic variation to traditional push-ups.

Incorporate wall push-up plus into your upper body workout routine for a challenging and effective exercise that contributes to a well-defined upper body.

To your strength and success

WALL PUSH UP

1. STARTING POSITION:

- Stand facing the wall, approximately arm's length away.

- Place your hands on the wall at shoulder height, slightly wider than shoulder-width apart.

- Ensure your feet are hip-width apart, creating a stable base.

2. BODY ALIGNMENT

- Maintain a straight line from your head to your heels.

- Engage your core muscles to keep your body in a plank-like position.

- Your arms should be fully extended, and your hands should be pressing into the wall.

3. DESCENT:

- Bend your elbows and lower your chest toward the wall.

- Keep your body in a straight line without letting your hips sag.

- Lower your chest until it almost touches the wall, maintaining control throughout the movement.

4. ASCENT:

- Push through your palms to extend your arms and return to the starting position.

- Fully straighten your elbows at the top of the movement.

- Focus on using your chest and arms to perform the push-up.

5. REPETITION:

Perform the desired number of repetitions, keeping a steady and controlled pace. If you're a beginner, start with a manageable number of reps and gradually increase as you build strength.

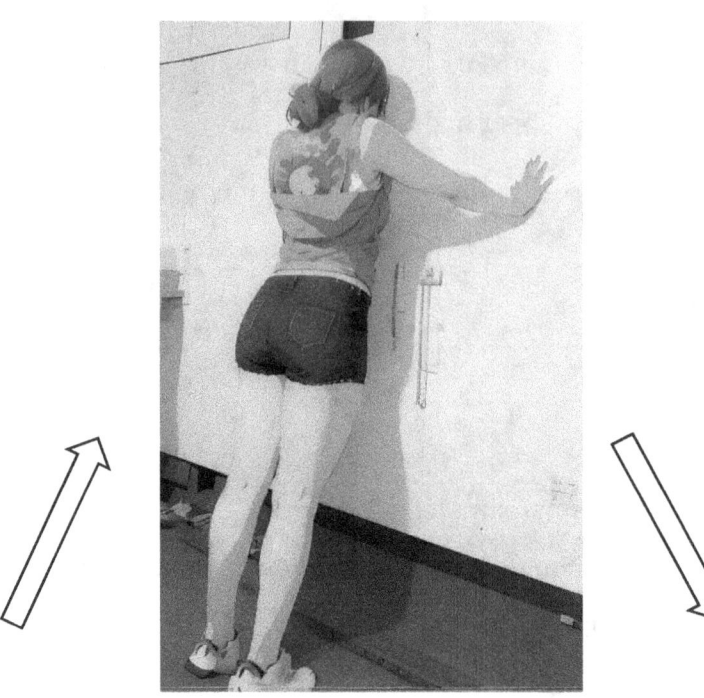

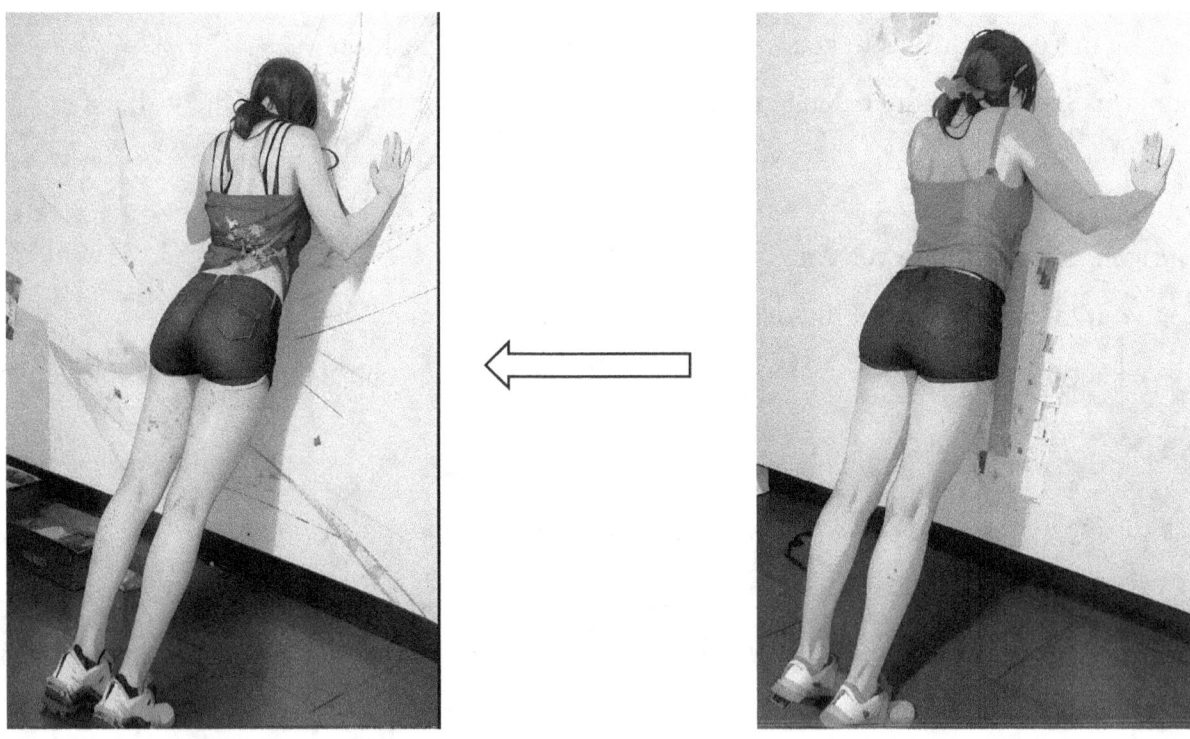

TIPS:

- Focus on controlled movements to maximize muscle engagement.
- Keep your neck in a neutral position, looking at the wall or slightly down.
- Maintain proper breathing throughout the exercise, exhaling during the push-up and inhaling during the ascent.

BENEFITS:

- Strengthens the chest, shoulders, and triceps.
- Builds upper body endurance.
- Beginner-friendly and accessible for individuals with limited mobility.

Incorporate wall push-ups into your routine to build upper body strength and gradually progress to more advanced variations. Whether you're a beginner or looking for a modification, wall push-ups are a versatile exercise for achieving upper body fitness.

To your strength and progress

FLOOR PUSH UP

1. STARTING POSITION:

- Begin in a prone position on the floor, facing down.
- Place your hands on the floor slightly wider than shoulder-width apart.
- Extend your legs straight, toes pointing towards the ground.
- Keep your body in a straight line from head to heels.

2. CORE ENGAGEMENT:

Engage your core muscles by pulling your navel towards your spine. Maintain a neutral spine throughout the movement.

3. DESCENT PHASE:

- Lower your body towards the floor by bending your elbows.

- Keep your elbows close to your body, not flaring outwards.
- Lower until your chest almost touches the floor.

4. ASCENT PHASE:

- Push through your palms to extend your arms, lifting your body back to the starting position.
- Fully extend your arms at the top, without locking your elbows.
- Ensure a smooth, controlled motion throughout the push-up.

5. BREATHING

- Inhale as you lower your body towards the floor.
- Exhale as you push back up to the starting position.

6. COMMON MISTAKES TO AVOID:

- Avoid sagging or arching your lower back; keep a straight line.
- Ensure your neck is in a neutral position, avoiding excessive tilting up or down.
- Maintain control throughout the movement; avoid using momentum.

7. MODIFICATIONS

- Perform push-ups on your knees if the standard variation is challenging.
- Elevate your hands on an elevated surface to reduce difficulty.

8. REPETITIONS:

Aim for a specific number of repetitions based on your fitness level. Gradually increase the reps as you build strength and endurance.

BENEFITS:

- Targets the chest, shoulders, and triceps.
- Engages the core for stability.
- Promotes upper body strength and muscle development.

Incorporate floor push-ups into your routine to build upper body strength and enhance overall fitness. Start with a manageable number of repetitions and gradually progress as you become more comfortable with the exercise.

To a stronger and fitter you.

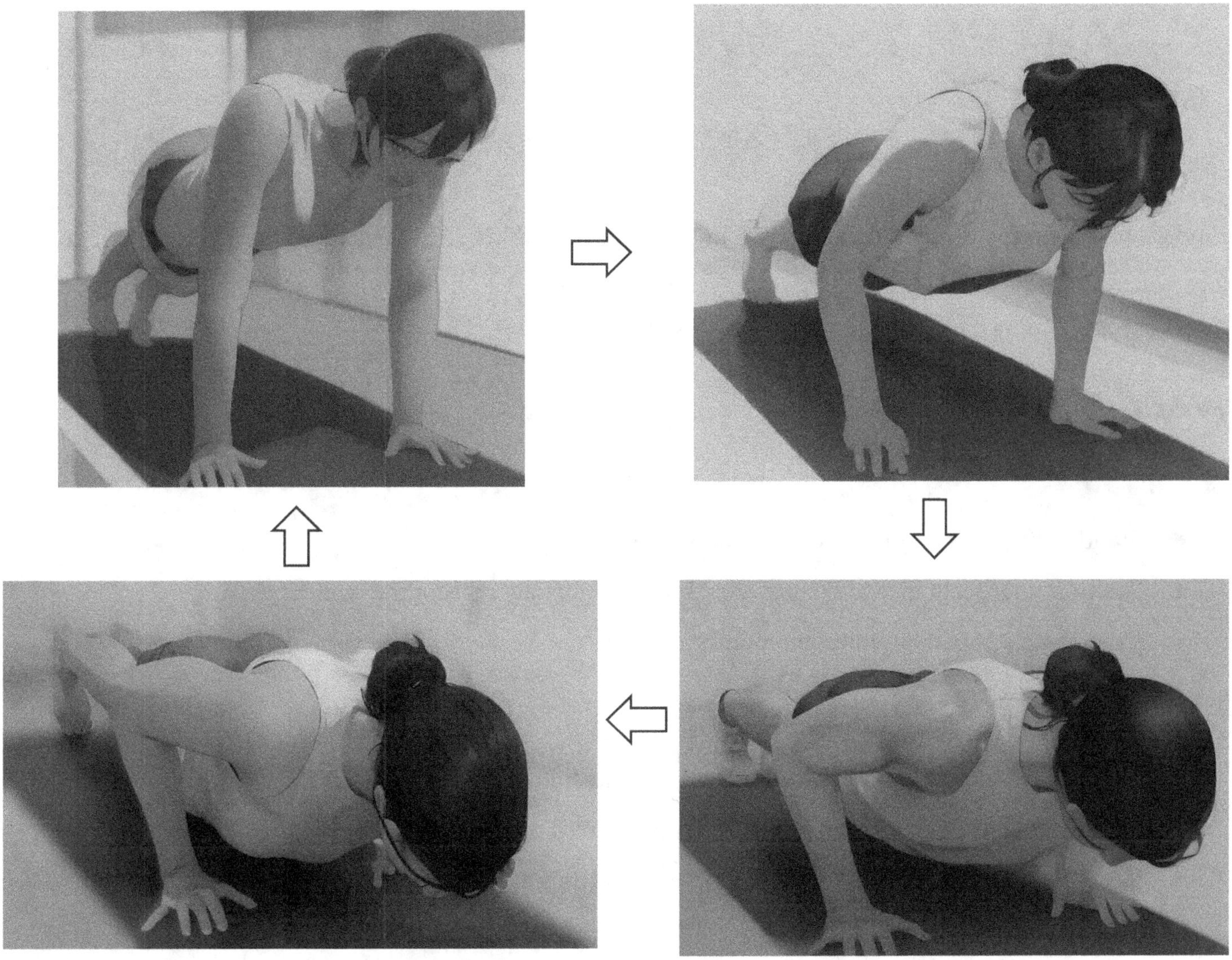

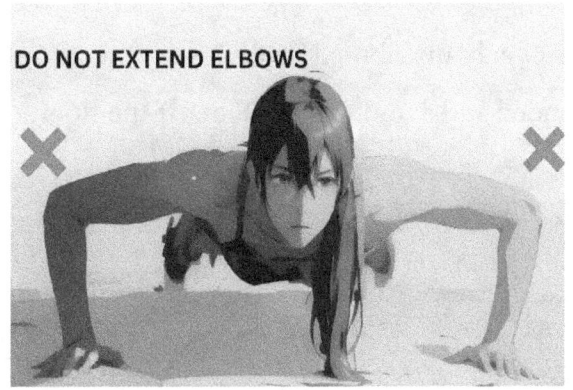

DO NOT EXTEND ELBOWS

CHAPTER 7 - LOWER BODY EXERCISES: SHAPE & DEFINE YOUR LOWER BODY

Embark on a journey to sculpt and define your lower body with these targeted exercises. Strengthen your legs, tone your glutes, and enhance overall lower body aesthetics. Follow the instructions below to perform each exercise with proper form and effectiveness.

WALL SQUAT HOLDS

1. STARTING POSITION

- Stand with your back against a flat and sturdy wall.
- Position your feet hip-width apart and about two feet away from the wall.
- Keep your feet parallel to each other.

2. DESCENT PHASE:

- Slowly lower your body by bending your knees, sliding down the wall.
- Aim for a seated position, ensuring your knees are directly above your ankles.
- Keep your back against the wall and maintain a straight posture.

3. THIGH POSITION:

- Ideally, your thighs should be parallel to the ground.
- If possible, lower yourself until your knees are at a 90-degree angle.

4. FOOT PLACEMENT:

- Ensure your weight is evenly distributed on both feet.
- Keep your heels grounded and avoid lifting them off the floor.

5. UPPER BODY ALIGNMENT:

Maintain a neutral spine with your back flat against the wall. Avoid leaning forward or rounding your back.

6. ARM POSITION:

- Place your hands on your hips or extend them straight in front of you for balance.
- Adjust your arm position based on comfort and stability.

7. HOLDING TIME:

Hold the squat position for a designated duration. Beginners may start with 15-30 seconds and progress over time.

8. BREATHING:

- Inhale deeply as you lower into the squat position.
- Exhale steadily to maintain control throughout the hold.

9. REPETITIONS AND SETS:

- Wall squat holds can be performed for a set duration or specific repetitions.
- Begin with a manageable time frame and gradually increase as you build strength.

10. COMMON MISTAKES TO AVOID:

- Ensure your knees stay aligned with your ankles, avoiding inward collapse.
- Watch for proper lower back alignment against the wall.
- Maintain control; avoid rapid descents or bouncing in the squat.

11. PROGRESSION:

As you gain strength, challenge yourself by holding the position for a longer time. Gradually increase the difficulty by incorporating variations or adding resistance.

BENEFITS:

- Strengthens quadriceps, hamstrings, and glutes.
- Improves lower body endurance.

- Enhances overall lower body stability.

Incorporate wall squat holds into your routine to shape and define your lower body. Whether you're a beginner or advanced fitness enthusiast, this exercise offers a versatile way to build strength and endurance in the lower body muscles.

To strong and sculpted legs. 🦵 💯

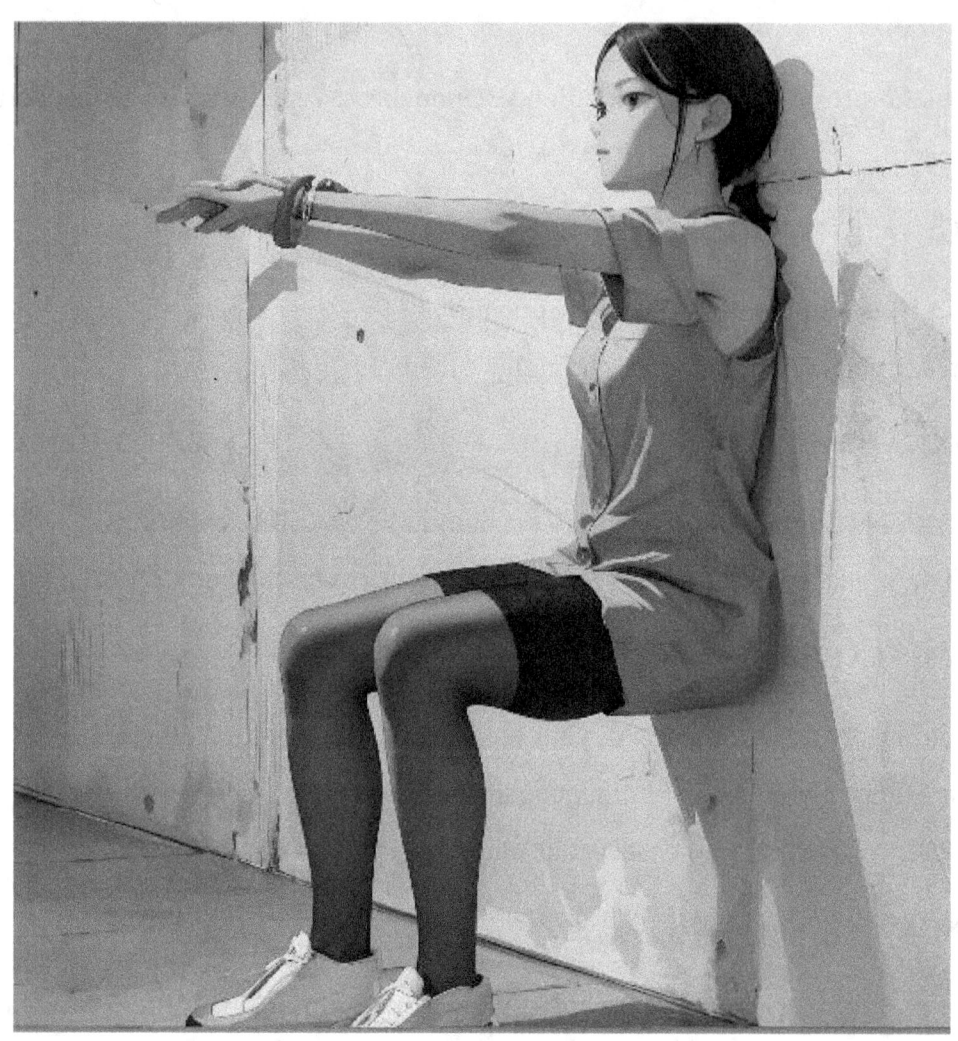

ELEVATED WALL LUNGES

Elevated wall lunges are an effective lower body exercise that targets the muscles of the legs and glutes. Follow these step-by-step instructions to ensure proper form and maximize the benefits of this exercise.

1. SETTING UP:

- Position yourself facing the wall with your feet hip-width apart.
- Place one foot behind you on an elevated surface such as a step or sturdy platform.
- Ensure the elevated foot is secure and stable.

2. BODY ALIGNMENT:

- Maintain a straight line from your head to your heels.
- Engage your core muscles to stabilize your spine.

3. DESCENT PHASE:

Lower your body by bending your front knee, ensuring it stays directly above your ankle. Simultaneously, allow your back knee to bend towards the ground.

4. DEEPEN THE LUNGE:

- Lower your body until your front thigh is parallel to the ground or as far as your flexibility allows.
- Ensure both knees are at approximately 90-degree angles.

5. ASCENT PHASE:

- Push through the heel of your front foot to return to the starting position.
- Extend both knees fully without locking them.

6. REPEAT ON THE OPPOSITE LEG:

- After completing the desired number of repetitions on one leg, switch to the other leg.
- Follow the same steps to perform elevated wall lunges on the opposite side.

7. BREATHING:

- Inhale as you lower your body into the lunge.
- Exhale as you push back up to the starting position.

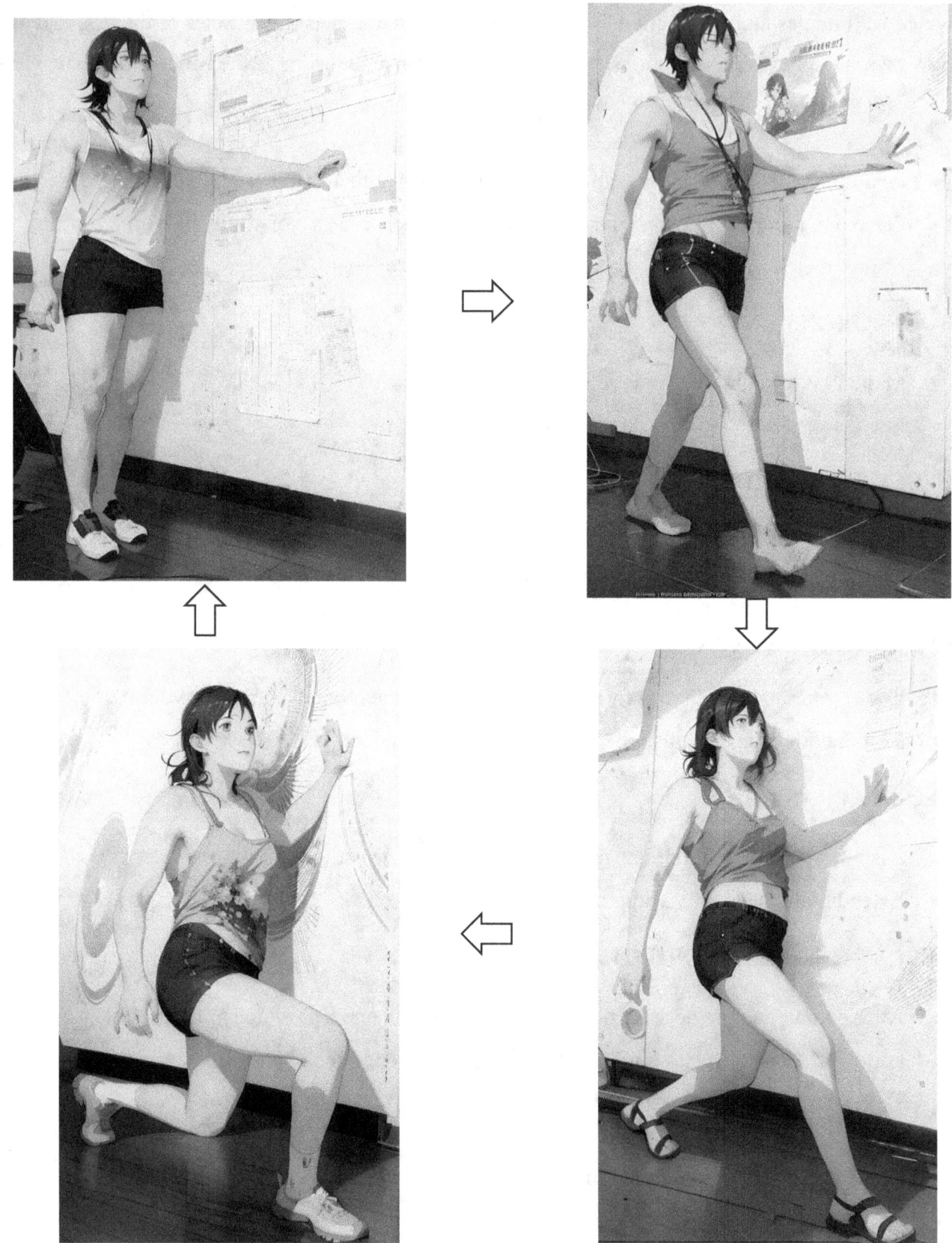

8. COMMON MISTAKES TO AVOID:

- Avoid leaning too far forward; maintain an upright torso.
- Ensure your front knee does not go beyond your toes during the descent.
- Keep your movements controlled to prevent any loss of balance.

9. REPETITIONS:

- Begin with a moderate number of repetitions, such as 10-12 on each leg.
- Adjust based on your fitness level and gradually increase as needed.

WALL-SUPPORTED PISTOL SQUATS

1. STARTING POSITION:

Stand facing the wall with your feet hip-width apart. Place your hands on the wall at shoulder height for support.

2. LIFTING ONE LEG:

- Shift your weight onto one leg and lift the opposite foot off the ground.
- Extend the lifted leg forward, keeping it straight or with a slight bend in the knee.

3. DESCENT PHASE:

- Begin lowering your body down by bending the knee of the supporting leg.
- Keep your back straight and chest up during the descent.
- Aim to lower your body as close to a seated position as possible.

4. ASCENT PHASE:

- Push through the heel of the supporting leg to rise back to the starting position.
- Straighten the supporting leg completely at the top of the movement.

5. REPEAT ON THE OTHER LEG:

Shift your weight to the opposite leg and repeat the exercise on the other side.

6. KEY POINTS:

- Maintain a neutral spine throughout the movement.
- Keep the knee of the supporting leg in line with the toes.
- Engage your core for stability.
- Control the movement to avoid momentum.

7. COMMON MISTAKES TO AVOID:

- Avoid rounding your back or leaning too far forward.
- Ensure the lifted leg is extended and controlled throughout the exercise.
- Focus on controlled movements rather than speed.

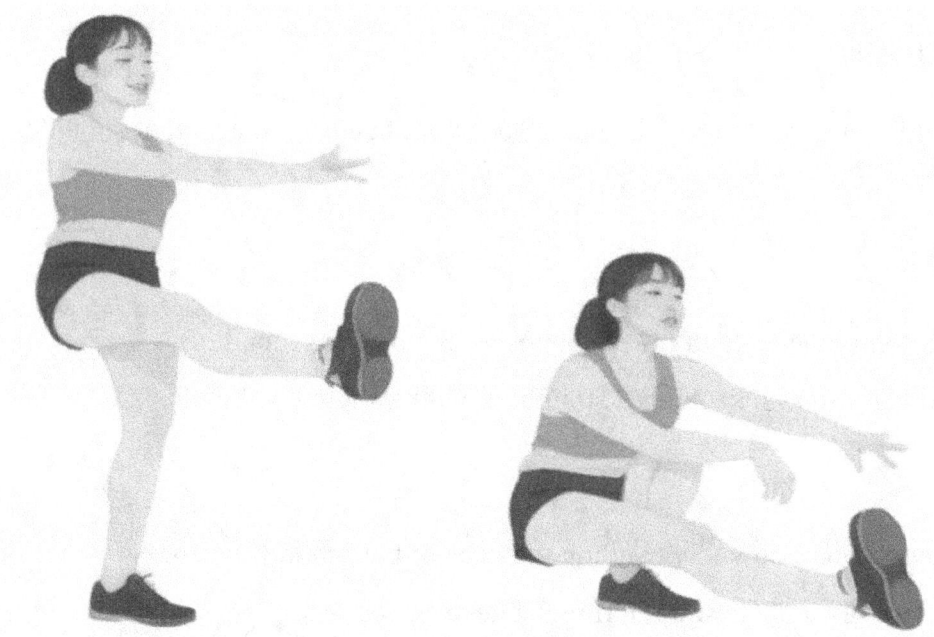

8. REPETITIONS:

- Aim for a specific number of repetitions on each leg, based on your fitness level.
- Gradually increase the reps as you build strength and stability.

BENEFITS:

- Targets the muscles of the lower body, including quads, hamstrings, and glutes.
- Improves balance and stability.
- Enhances overall lower body strength and flexibility.

GLUTE BRIDGE WALL SLIDES

Elevate your lower body workout with the glute bridge wall slides, a dynamic exercise that engages your glutes, hamstrings, and hip flexors.

1. STARTING POSITION:

- Lie on your back with your feet flat on the ground, hip-width apart.
- Place your arms by your sides with palms facing down.
- Ensure your spine is in a neutral position, maintaining a natural curve in your lower back.

2. GLUTE BRIDGE:

- Press through your heels to lift your hips up.
- Squeeze your glutes at the top of the bridge to fully engage your posterior chain.
- Maintain a straight line from shoulders to knees at the peak of the bridge.

3. WALL SLIDES:

- While holding the glute bridge position, slide one foot up the wall.
- Keep the knee bent at a 90-degree angle, bringing the thigh parallel to the ground.
- Slide the foot back down to the starting position, maintaining the bridge.
- Alternate legs and repeat the sliding motion.

4. BREATHING:

- Inhale as you lift your hips into the glute bridge position.
- Exhale as you perform the sliding motion.

5. CORE ENGAGEMENT:

Keep your core muscles engaged throughout the exercise to stabilize your spine.

6. REPETITIONS:

Aim for a specific number of repetitions on each leg.

Gradually increase the reps as your strength and stability improve.

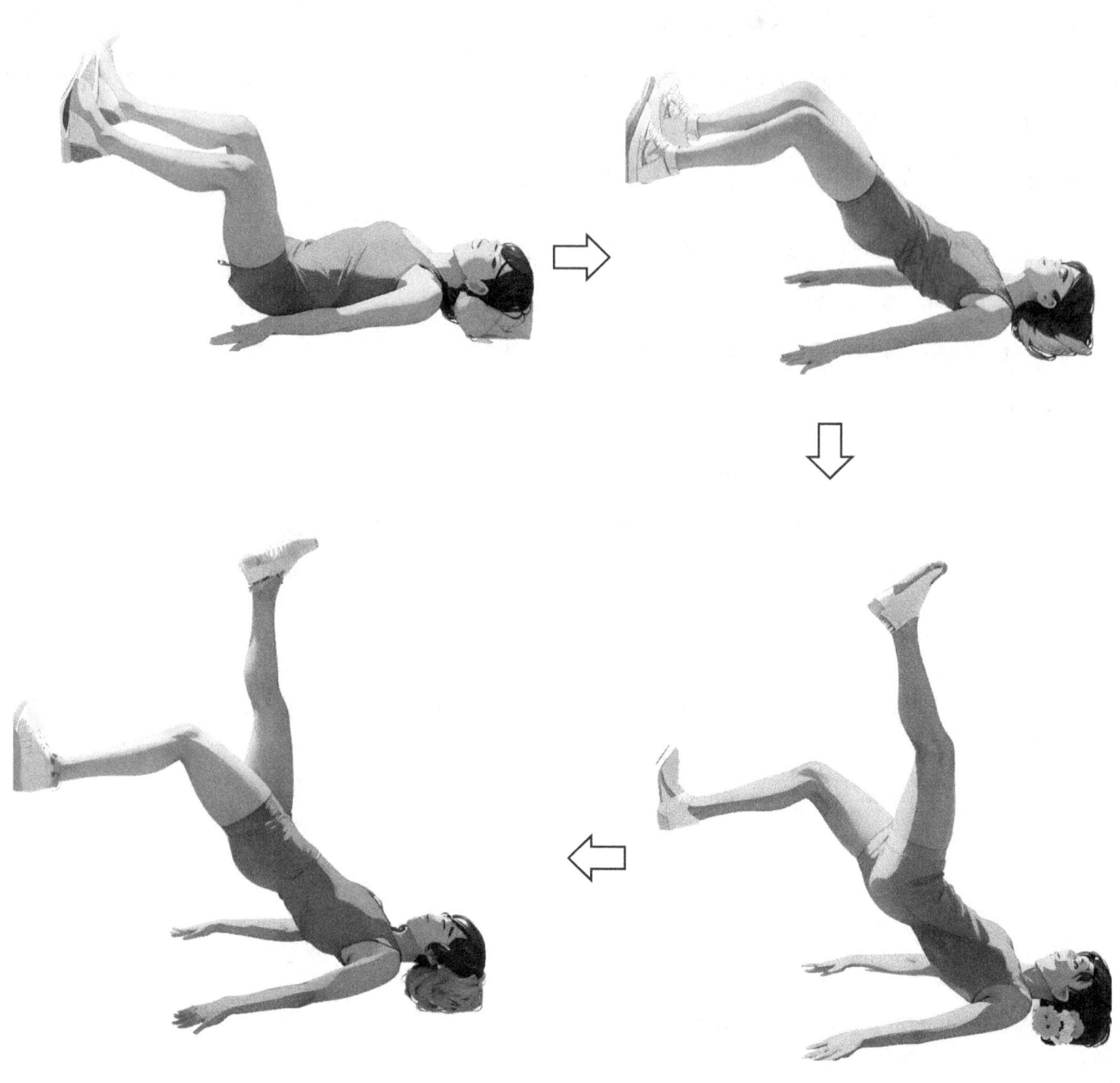

7. COMMON MISTAKES TO AVOID:

- Avoid overarching your lower back during the glute bridge.
- Ensure both hips stay level during the sliding motion.
- Maintain control to prevent excessive swinging or instability.

BENEFITS:

- Targets and activates the glutes, hamstrings, and hip flexors.
- Enhances hip mobility and stability.
- Strengthens the posterior chain for improved athletic performance.

Incorporate glute bridge wall slides into your lower body routine for a challenging and effective workout. This exercise not only shapes your glutes but also promotes overall lower body strength and stability.

Happy sliding and strengthening! 🏋️

WALL SIDE LEG LIFTS

Wall side leg lifts are effective for targeting the outer thighs and hips. Follow these step-by-step instructions to perform this exercise with proper form and maximize its benefits.

1. STARTING POSITION:

Stand with your side facing the wall, placing one hand on the wall for support. Keep your feet together and your core engaged.

2. LEG LIFT:

- Lift your outer leg to the side, keeping it straight.
- Focus on using the muscles on the outer part of your hip and thigh.
- Lift your leg as high as comfortably possible without compromising your form.

3. CONTROLLED LOWERING:

- Slowly lower your leg back to the starting position.
- Maintain control throughout the lowering phase to engage the muscles effectively.

4. REPETITIONS:

- Perform the desired number of repetitions on one leg before switching to the other.
- Aim for a controlled and deliberate movement to maximize the benefits.

5. BREATHING:

Inhale as you lift your leg. Exhale as you lower your leg.

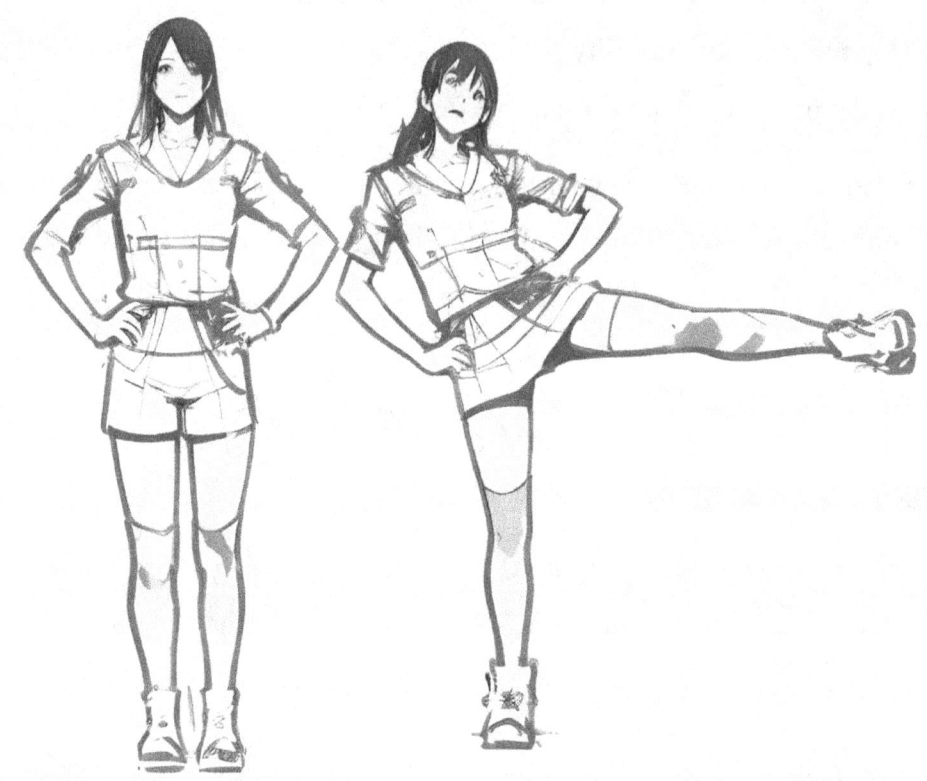

6. TIPS:

- Keep your core engaged to stabilize your body.
- Avoid leaning too much on the supporting hand; use it for balance rather than support.
- Focus on the outer part of your hip and thigh to target the intended muscles.

7. MODIFICATIONS:

- If needed, perform the exercise close to a wall for additional support.
- Adjust the height of your leg lift based on your comfort and fitness level.

Incorporate wall side leg lifts into your lower body workout routine to strengthen and tone the outer thighs and hips. This exercise contributes to a well-rounded lower body workout, helping you achieve balance and definition in this key area.

To a stronger and more sculpted you.

WALL SQUAT WITH CALF RAISE

Wall squat with calf raise targets your quads, hamstrings, glutes, and calves, providing a comprehensive lower body workout. Follow these steps to perform the exercise with proper form and effectiveness.

1. STARTING POSITION:

- Stand with your back against the wall, ensuring it provides support for your entire spine.
- Position your feet shoulder-width apart, a comfortable distance from the wall.
- Engage your core muscles for stability.

2. WALL SQUAT PHASE:

- Lower your body into a squatting position by bending your knees.
- Slide down the wall while maintaining contact with your back.
- Keep your knees directly above your ankles, avoiding inward collapsing.

3. CALF RAISE PHASE:

- Once in the squat position, push through your heels to rise onto the balls of your feet.
- Lift your heels off the ground, engaging your calf muscles.
- Hold the raised position for a moment to maximize the calf contraction.

4. DESCENT AND REPEAT:

- Lower your heels back to the ground, returning to the initial squat position.
- Ensure a controlled descent, maintaining stability against the wall.
- Repeat the sequence for the desired number of repetitions.

5. BREATHING:

- Inhale as you descend into the wall squat.

- Exhale as you push through your heels to perform the calf raise.

6. COMMON MISTAKES TO AVOID:

- Avoid letting your knees collapse inward during the squat phase.

- Maintain a smooth, controlled motion without jerking movements.

- Ensure your back stays in contact with the wall throughout the exercise.

7. BENEFITS:

- Targets quads, hamstrings, glutes, and calves.

- Enhances lower body strength and endurance.

- Promotes stability and balance.

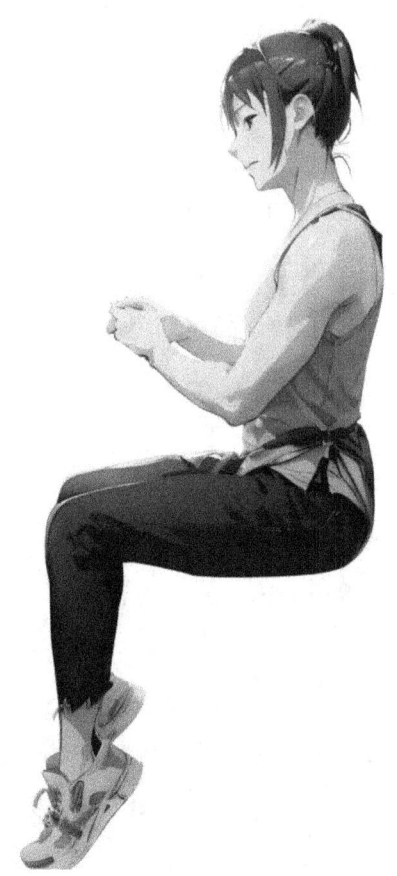

ELEVATED STALLION PULSES

Elevated stallion pulses are an effective exercise to target and sculpt your glutes and thighs. Follow these step-by-step instructions to ensure proper form and maximize the benefits of this lower body exercise.

1. STARTING POSITION:

- Stand facing the wall with your feet hip-width apart.
- Place your hands on the wall at shoulder height for support.
- Lift one leg and place the foot on an elevated surface behind you, creating a 90-degree angle with the knee.

2. ENGAGE YOUR CORE:

Tighten your core muscles to maintain stability throughout the movement.

3. PULSE MOTION:

- Lower your body into a partial squat by bending your standing leg.
- Perform small, controlled pulses by moving your body up and down within a short range of motion.
- Focus on engaging your glutes and thigh muscles during each pulse.

4. REPETITIONS:

Perform the pulses for a specified number of repetitions, gradually increasing as your strength improves. Switch to the other leg and repeat the exercise.

5. BREATHING:

Inhale as you lower your body into the pulse position. Exhale as you lift your body back to the starting position.

6. COMMON MISTAKES TO AVOID:

- Avoid leaning too heavily on the wall; use it for support without relying on it.
- Keep the standing knee aligned with the ankle to prevent strain on the knee joint.
- Maintain a controlled pace and avoid bouncing during the pulses.

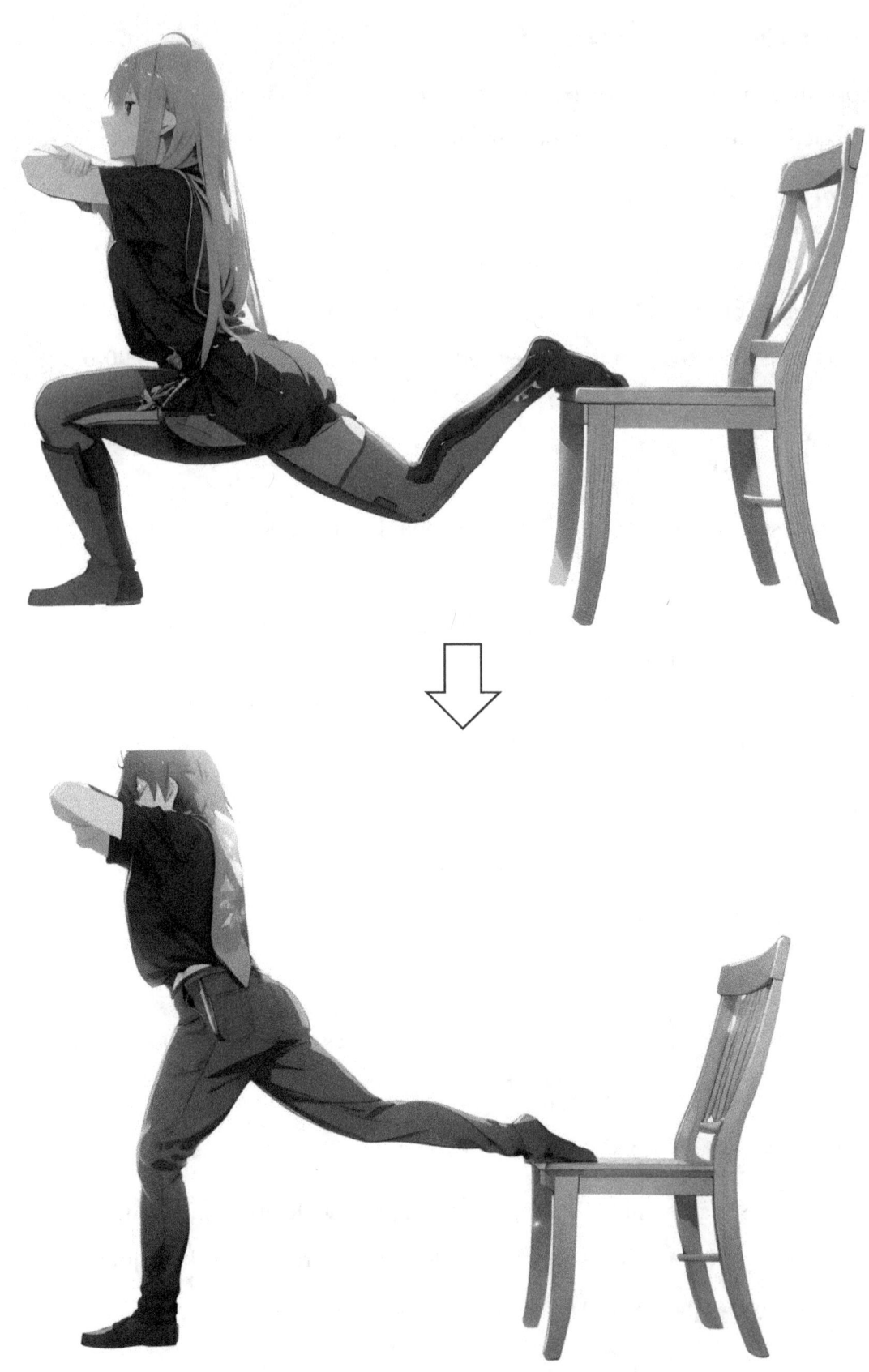

7. BENEFITS:

- Targets the glutes, thighs, and lower body muscles.
- Enhances muscle definition and toning.
- Helps improve balance and stability.

Incorporate elevated stallion pulses into your lower body workout routine to add variety and intensity. Adjust the difficulty by choosing an appropriate height for the elevated surface and gradually progressing as you build strength. Enjoy the burn as you work towards sculpting strong and shapely lower body muscles.

To a sculpted and toned you.

HIGH WALL GLUTE KICKBACKS

1. SETUP:

- Begin by standing facing the wall, with your hands placed on the wall at shoulder height.
- Your arms should be fully extended, and your feet hip-width apart.
- Engage your core for stability throughout the exercise.

2. KICKBACK MOVEMENT:

- Lift your right leg straight back, keeping it in line with your body.
- Focus on using your glute muscles to lift the leg, avoiding excessive arching in your lower back.
- Squeeze your glutes at the top of the movement to fully engage the muscles.

3. LOWERING PHASE:

- Bring your right leg back down in a controlled manner, returning to the starting position.
- Maintain a slow and controlled pace to maximize muscle activation.

4. REPETITIONS:

Perform the desired number of repetitions on one leg before switching to the other. Aim for a smooth and controlled movement throughout each repetition.

5. BREATHING:

- Inhale as you lift your leg.
- Exhale as you lower your leg back down.

6. COMMON MISTAKES TO AVOID:

- Avoid overarching your lower back; keep your spine neutral.
- Ensure your hips remain squared to the wall throughout the movement.
- Focus on isolating the glutes; minimize involvement of the lower back.

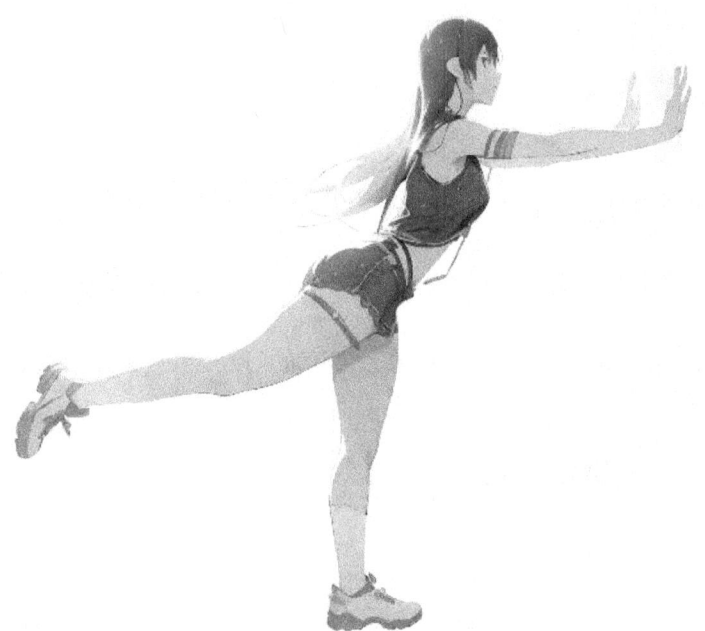

7. MODIFICATIONS:

- If needed, perform the exercise with a smaller range of motion until you build strength and stability.
- Adjust the distance from the wall based on your comfort and balance.

8. BENEFITS:

- Targets and sculpts the glute muscles.
- Enhances hip stability and strength.
- Can help improve overall lower body aesthetics.

HIP FLEXOR MARCH.

1. STARTING POSITION:

- Stand with your feet hip-width apart.
- Ensure your posture is upright, shoulders back, and core engaged.

2. RAISE ONE KNEE:

- Lift your right knee towards your chest, engaging your hip flexors.
- Keep the movement controlled and deliberate.
- Maintain a straight posture; avoid leaning backward or forward.

3. HOLD AND LOWER:

- Hold your right knee in the raised position for a moment, emphasizing the contraction.
- Lower the right foot back to the starting position.
- Ensure a smooth and controlled descent.

4. ALTERNATE LEGS:

- Repeat the same movement with your left leg, lifting the knee towards your chest.
- Hold and lower the left foot back to the starting position.

5. CONTINUED MARCHING:

- Continue alternating between right and left legs, creating a marching motion.
- Aim for a rhythmic and controlled pace throughout the exercise.

6. BREATHING:

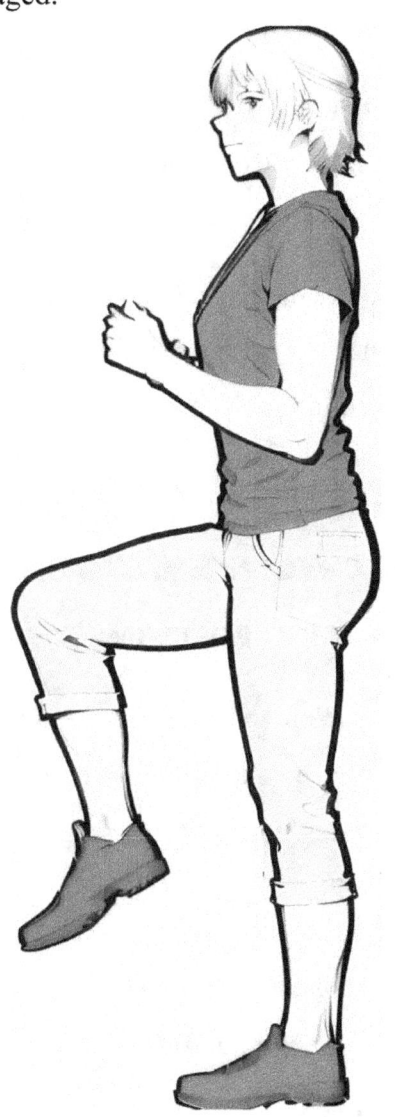

Inhale as you lift one knee towards your chest. Exhale as you lower the foot back to the ground.

7. COMMON MISTAKES TO AVOID:

- Avoid lifting the knee too high, maintaining a comfortable range of motion.
- Keep your core engaged to prevent excessive arching or rounding of the lower back.
- Ensure your shoulders remain relaxed; avoid shrugging.

8. BENEFITS:

- Targets the hip flexors, thighs, and core muscles.
- Improves hip flexibility and range of motion.
- Enhances overall lower body mobility.

Incorporate the hip flexor march into your routine to promote flexibility and strength in the hip region. Start with a moderate pace and gradually increase intensity as your muscles adapt. Enjoy the benefits of improved hip mobility.

WALL GLUTE BRIDGE.

1. STARTING POSITION:

- Lie on your back on the floor with your feet flat against the wall.
- Place your feet hip-width apart and about a foot away from the wall.
- Keep your arms by your sides, palms facing down.

2. CORE ENGAGEMENT:

- Engage your core by pulling your navel towards your spine.
- Ensure a neutral spine with a slight natural curve in your lower back.

3. HIP LIFT:

- Press through your heels to lift your hips towards the ceiling.
- Focus on squeezing your glutes at the top of the movement.
- Your body should form a straight line from shoulders to knees at the peak.

4. LOWERING PHASE:

- Lower your hips back down towards the floor with control.
- Avoid letting your back arch excessively during the descent.
- Allow your hips to lightly touch the floor before lifting again.

5. BREATHING:

- Inhale as you prepare to lift your hips.
- Exhale as you lift your hips towards the ceiling.
- Inhale as you lower your hips back down.

6. REPETITIONS:

- Aim for a specific number of repetitions based on your fitness level.
- Increase the reps gradually as your strength improves.

7. COMMON MISTAKES TO AVOID

- Avoid pushing through your toes; focus on heel drive.
- Ensure your knees stay in line with your hips during the lift.
- Keep your neck and shoulders relaxed throughout the movement.

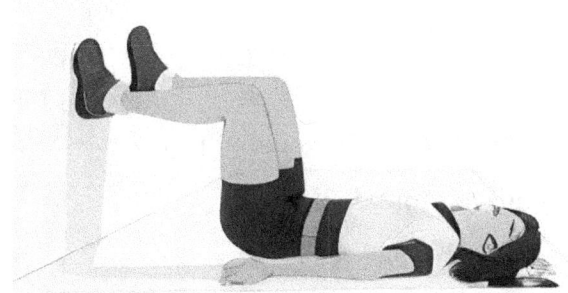 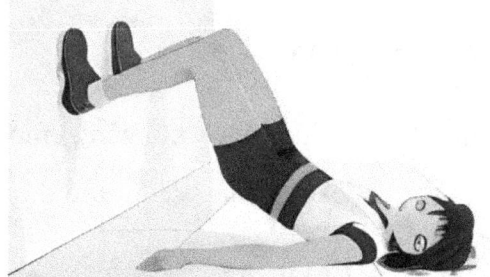

8. BENEFITS:

- Targets and activates the glutes, hamstrings, and lower back.
- Improves lower body strength and stability.
- Enhances overall lower body muscle tone.

Incorporate the wall glute bridge into your routine to build strength and definition in your lower body. It's a versatile exercise suitable for various fitness levels, offering an effective way to sculpt your glutes and improve lower body functionality.

Enjoy the journey to a stronger and more toned lower body! 🏋️

WALL FIRE HYDRANT

1. STARTING POSITION:

Stand facing the wall, with your hands placed firmly on the wall at shoulder height. Maintain a straight alignment from head to heels.

2. LIFTING LEG TO THE SIDE:

- Lift your right leg out to the side, keeping the knee bent at a 90-degree angle.
- Focus on engaging your glutes and outer thigh muscles during the lift.
- Keep the movement controlled and avoid swinging the leg.

3. PEAK CONTRACTION

- Hold the lifted position for a moment, emphasizing the contraction in the glutes.
- Ensure your pelvis remains stable, and the core is engaged for balance.

4. LOWERING THE LEG:

- Gently lower your right leg back to the starting position.
- Control the descent to work the muscles eccentrically.

5. REPEAT ON THE OTHER LEG:

Perform the same sequence with your left leg to ensure balanced muscle development.

6. BREATHING:

Inhale as you lift your leg to the side. Exhale as you lower the leg back to the starting position.

7. COMMON MISTAKES TO AVOID:

- Avoid leaning excessively towards the wall; keep your upper body stable.
- Maintain a controlled pace, avoiding rapid or jerky movements.
- Focus on the abduction of the hip rather than rotation.

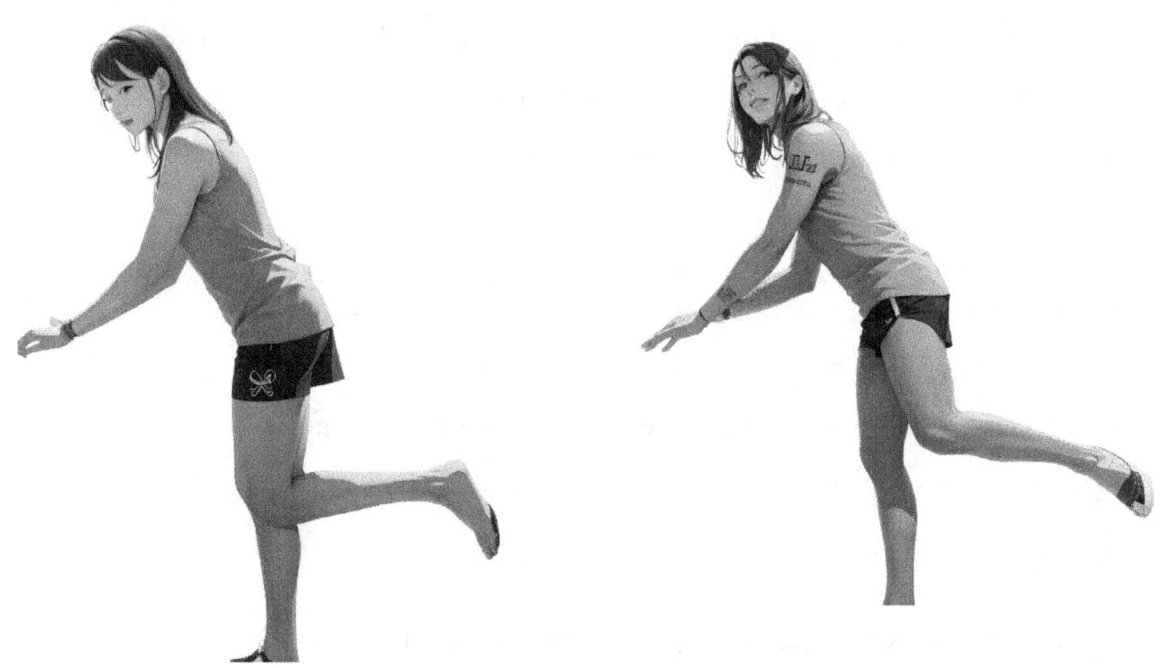

8. REPETITIONS:

Aim for a specific number of repetitions on each leg based on your fitness level. Gradually increase the reps as you build strength and control.

BENEFITS:

- Targets the glutes, particularly the gluteus medius.
- Enhances hip abduction strength and stability.
- Can help improve overall lower body aesthetics.

Integrate the wall fire hydrant into your lower body workout routine to add variety and target specific muscle groups. Remember to perform the exercise in a controlled manner, focusing on the mind-muscle connection for optimal results.

To a sculpted and strong lower body ✦

WALL COSSACK SQUAT

- **STARTING POSITION:**
- Stand with your back against the wall, feet slightly wider than shoulder-width apart.
- Place your hands on the wall for support at shoulder height.
- Ensure your feet are parallel to each other or slightly turned outward.

2. DESCENT PHASE:

- Shift your weight to one side as you bend the knee of that leg.
- Simultaneously, straighten the opposite leg, extending it to the side.
- Lower your body towards the bent knee, keeping your back straight.
- Go as low as your flexibility allows, aiming for a deep squat position.

3. ASCENT PHASE:

- Push through the heel of the bent leg to return to the starting position.
- Simultaneously, bring the extended leg back to the center.

4. REPEAT ON THE OTHER SIDE:

- Perform the Cossack Squat on the opposite side by shifting your weight to the other leg.
- Maintain a controlled and fluid motion throughout the exercise.

5. BREATHING:

Inhale as you descend into the squat position. Exhale as you push back up to the starting position.

6. COMMON MISTAKES TO AVOID:

- Ensure your knee is aligned with your toes during the descent to protect the joint.

- Keep your back straight and chest lifted throughout the movement.
- Maintain stability; avoid excessive leaning or tilting.

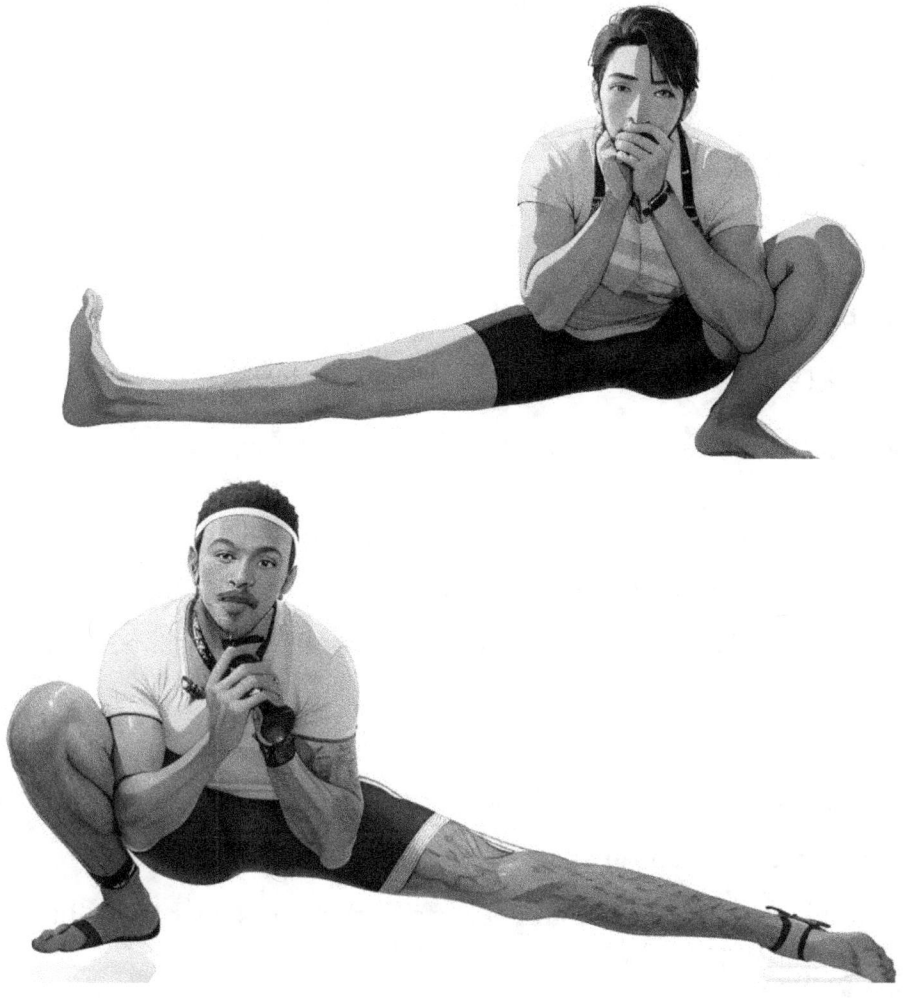

7. FLEXIBILITY AND STRENGTH BENEFITS:

- Increases flexibility in the hips and thighs.
- Strengthens the quadriceps, hamstrings, and glutes.
- Improves balance and stability.

8. REPETITIONS:

- Begin with a moderate number of repetitions and gradually increase as you become more comfortable with the exercise.
- Aim for 2-3 sets with 10-15 repetitions on each side.

Incorporate the Wall Cossack Squat into your lower body workout routine to enhance flexibility, strength, and overall lower body functionality. As with any exercise, start at a level that suits your fitness ability and progress gradually. Enjoy the journey to a stronger and more flexible you!

WALL-FACING SQUAT

1. STARTING POSITION:

- Stand with your feet about hip-width apart.
- Ensure your feet are a comfortable distance away from the wall, allowing for a full range of motion.

2. HAND PLACEMENT:

- Extend your arms forward at shoulder height, parallel to the ground.
- Place your palms on the wall, shoulder-width apart.
- Your hands will help with balance and stability throughout the exercise.

3. SQUAT DESCENT:

- Lower your body into a squat position by bending your knees.
- Keep your back straight, chest up, and core engaged.
- Aim to bring your thighs parallel to the ground, or as far down as your flexibility allows.

4. ALIGNMENT AND FORM:

- Ensure your knees are directly above your ankles during the squat.
- Your weight should be evenly distributed through your heels and midfoot.
- Maintain a neutral spine throughout the movement.

5. ENGAGE MUSCLES:

Focus on engaging your quadriceps, hamstrings, and glutes as you push through your heels to return to the starting position.

Squeeze your glutes at the top of the movement for added engagement.

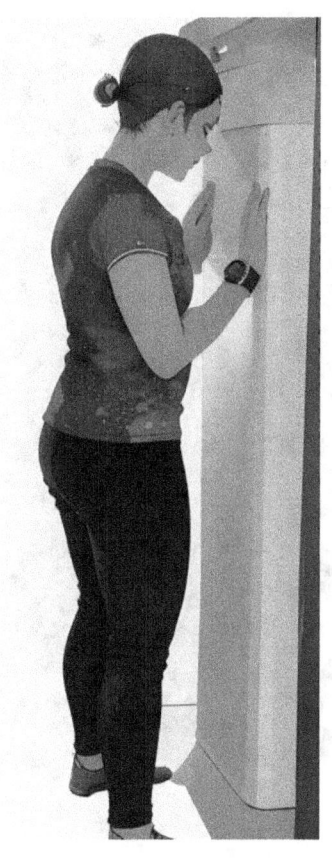
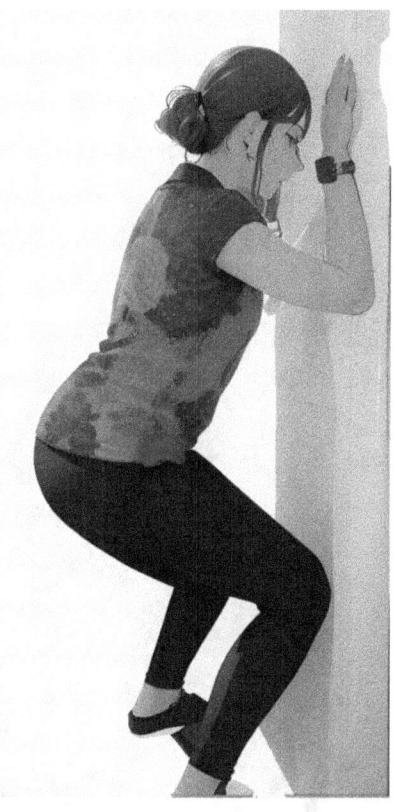

6. BREATHING:

Inhale as you descend into the squat. Exhale as you push back up to the starting position.

7. REPETITIONS:

Perform the wall-facing squat for a specific number of repetitions, depending on your fitness level. Gradually increase the reps as you become more comfortable with the exercise.

8. BENEFITS:

- Targets the quadriceps, hamstrings, glutes, and calves.
- Builds lower body strength and endurance.
- Enhances overall lower body muscle tone.

Incorporate the wall-facing squat into your lower body workout routine to shape and strengthen key muscle groups. Remember to focus on proper form and alignment to maximize the benefits of this effective exercise.

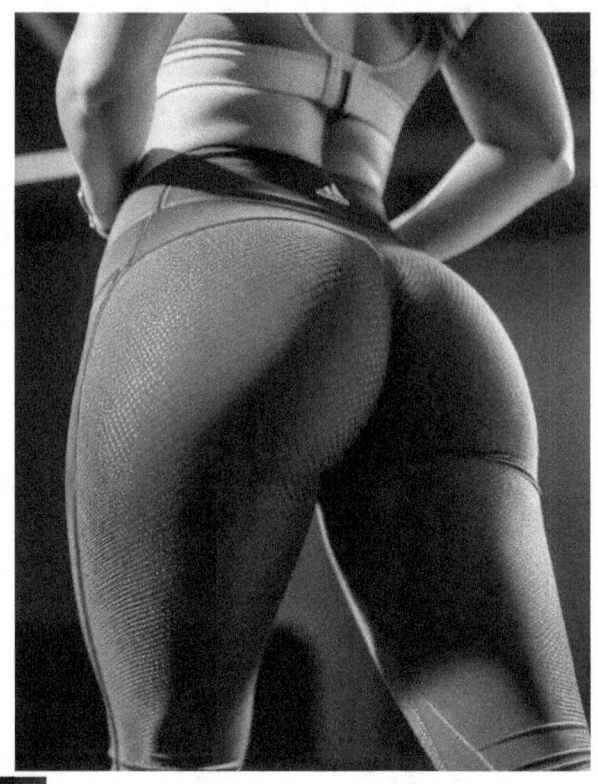

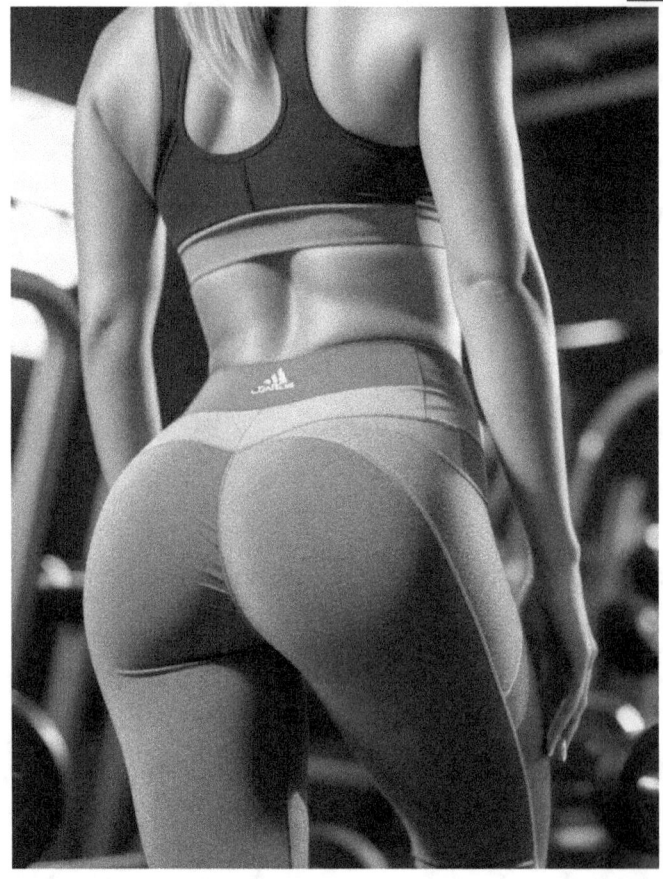

CHAPTER 8 - FLEXIBILITY & BALANCE EXERCISES

Improve your overall well-being by incorporating these balance and flexibility exercises into your routine. Enhance your stability, increase flexibility, and find a deeper connection with your body through the following exercises:

FLEXIBILITY

WALL FORWARD FOLD

1. SETUP:

Stand facing the wall with your feet hip-width apart. Ensure your toes are pointing forward and your heels are slightly away from the wall.

2. INITIATE THE FOLD:

Inhale deeply, lengthening your spine. Exhale as you hinge at your hips, reaching your hands towards the wall.

3. HAND PLACEMENT:

Place your hands on the wall at shoulder height, shoulder-width apart. Allow your head to hang between your arms.

4. LEG POSITION:

Keep a slight bend in your knees to avoid locking them. Engage your quadriceps to support the stretch.

5. HIP HINGE:

- Maintain a strong hip hinge as you fold forward.
- Feel the stretch in your hamstrings, lower back, and the back of your thighs.

6. RELAX INTO THE STRETCH:

- Allow your upper body to relax into the stretch.
- Breathe deeply and focus on releasing tension.

7. MODIFICATIONS:

- If flexibility allows, you can gradually straighten your legs for a deeper stretch.
- Adjust the distance between your feet and the wall based on your comfort level.

8. DURATION:

- Hold the stretch for 20-30 seconds, breathing deeply throughout.
- Gradually increase the duration as your flexibility improves.

9. EXITING THE STRETCH:

- Inhale as you slowly roll back up, stacking your spine vertebra by vertebra.
- Keep your movements controlled to prevent dizziness.

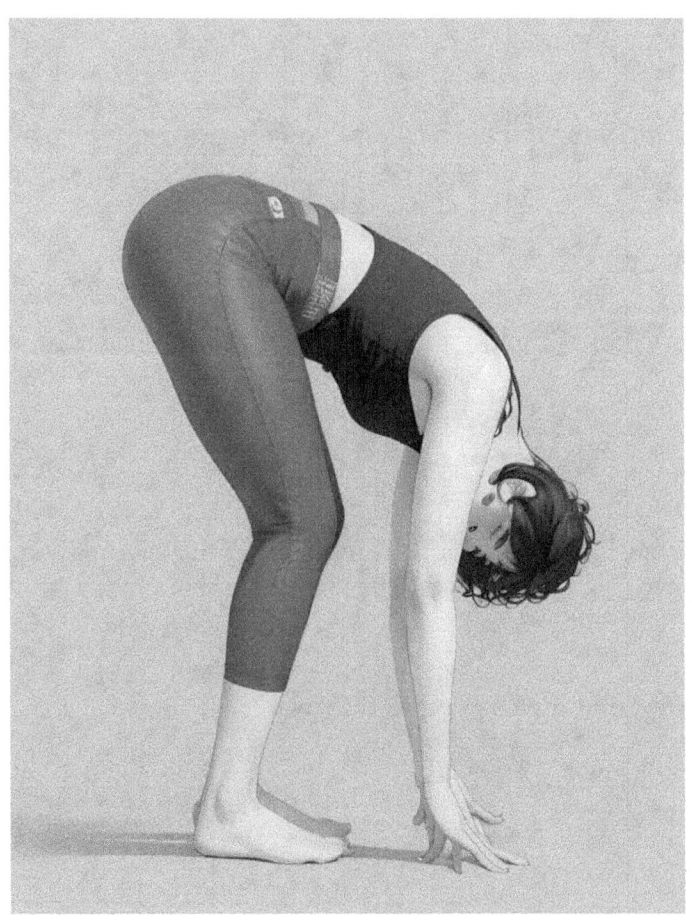

10. BENEFITS:

- Stretches the hamstrings, lower back, and calves.
- Promotes flexibility in the spine.
- Relieves tension in the upper back and shoulders.

11. CAUTION:

Avoid overstretching; only go as far as your body allows. If you have back issues, consult with a healthcare professional before attempting.

Incorporate the Wall Forward Fold into your routine for a rejuvenating stretch that targets key muscle groups. Enjoy the benefits of increased flexibility and a sense of relaxation as you make this stretch a regular part of your wellness practice.

WALL CHEST OPENER

1. STARTING POSITION:

- Stand facing the wall with your feet hip-width apart.
- Place your palms flat on the wall at shoulder height, fingers pointing upward.
- Keep your elbows slightly bent and in line with your shoulders.

2. ENGAGE YOUR CORE:

- Tighten your abdominal muscles to stabilize your spine.
- Ensure a neutral spine position with a straight back.

3. OPEN YOUR CHEST:

- Slowly lean your body forward, allowing your chest to move towards the wall.
- Keep your shoulders down and away from your ears.
- Focus on feeling a gentle stretch across your chest and the front of your shoulders.

4. BREATHING TECHNIQUE:

- Inhale deeply as you prepare for the stretch.

- Exhale gradually as you lean into the wall, deepening the chest opening.

5. HOLD THE STRETCH:

- Maintain the stretched position for 15-30 seconds, allowing your muscles to relax and lengthen.
- Avoid any bouncing or sudden movements; aim for a steady and controlled stretch.

6. RETURNING TO STARTING POSITION:

- Slowly push yourself away from the wall, bringing your body back to an upright position.
- Relax your arms by your sides.

7. REPEAT AS NEEDED:

Perform the Wall Chest Opener stretch for 2-3 repetitions, gradually increasing the duration as your flexibility improves.

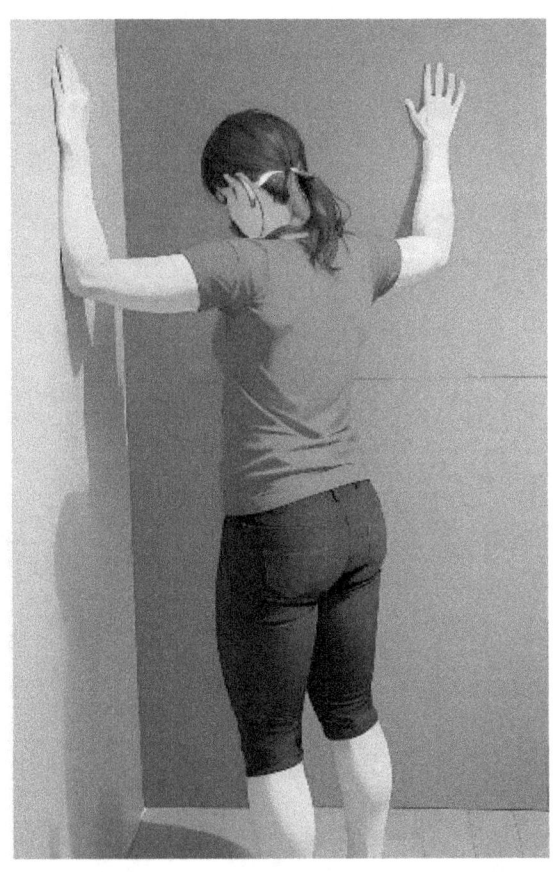 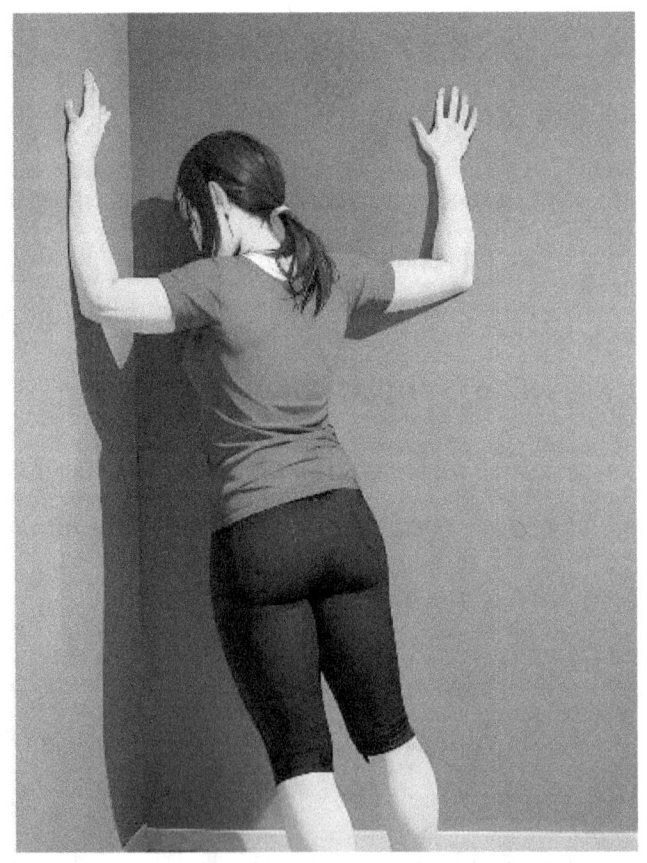

8. TIPS AND REMINDERS:

- Adjust the distance between your feet and the wall based on your comfort level.
- Modify the stretch intensity by altering the height of your hands on the wall.
- If you experience any discomfort or pain, ease off the stretch and consult with a fitness professional.

9. BENEFITS OF WALL CHEST OPENER:

- Releases tension in the chest and shoulders.
- Improves posture by counteracting the effects of hunching forward.
- Enhances flexibility in the chest muscles.

10. INCORPORATION INTO YOUR ROUTINE:

Include the Wall Chest Opener in your warm-up or cool-down routine. Pair it with other upper body stretches for a comprehensive flexibility session.

WALL TRICEP STRETCH

1. SETUP:

Stand facing a wall with your feet hip-width apart.

Extend your right arm straight, reaching towards the ceiling.

2. ARM PLACEMENT:

Bend your right elbow and bring your hand down your upper back.

Reach your left hand behind your back, aiming to touch your right elbow.

3. CONTACT WITH THE WALL:

Press your right palm against the wall with your fingers pointing down.

Keep your back straight and chest lifted throughout the stretch.

4. GENTLE PRESSURE:

Apply gentle pressure on your right elbow with your left hand to deepen the stretch.

Focus on feeling the stretch along the back of your right arm and triceps.

5. BREATHING:

Inhale deeply, expanding your chest.

Exhale slowly, allowing your muscles to relax into the stretch.

6. HOLDING THE STRETCH:

Hold the position for 15-30 seconds, allowing the triceps to release tension.

Maintain a comfortable stretch without any sharp pain.

7. SWITCH SIDES:

Repeat the stretch on the left arm by extending the left arm towards the ceiling and following the same steps.

8. BENEFITS:

Improves flexibility in the triceps and shoulders.

Alleviates tension in the upper arms.

Enhances overall upper body mobility.

WALL HIP FLEXOR STRETCH

1. POSITIONING:

Stand facing the wall with your feet hip-width apart. Place your hands on the wall at shoulder height for support.

2. STEP BACK:

- Take a step back with your right foot, keeping the toes pointing forward.
- Ensure your left foot remains closer to the wall.

3. LUNGE POSITION:

- Lower your body into a lunge, bending your left knee while keeping your right leg straight behind you.
- The back of your right heel should be on the ground.

4. HIP ALIGNMENT:

- Check that your hips are square and facing forward.
- You should feel a stretch in the front of your right hip, targeting the hip flexor.

5. UPPER BODY ALIGNMENT:

- Keep your upper body upright, with your spine in a neutral position.
- Avoid arching your back excessively; engage your core for stability.

6. HOLDING THE STRETCH:

- Hold the stretch for 20-30 seconds, focusing on deep and steady breaths.
- Feel the gentle release of tension in your hip flexors.

7. SWITCH SIDES:

- Return to the starting position and switch to stretch the left hip flexor.
- Repeat the same steps, ensuring proper form and alignment.

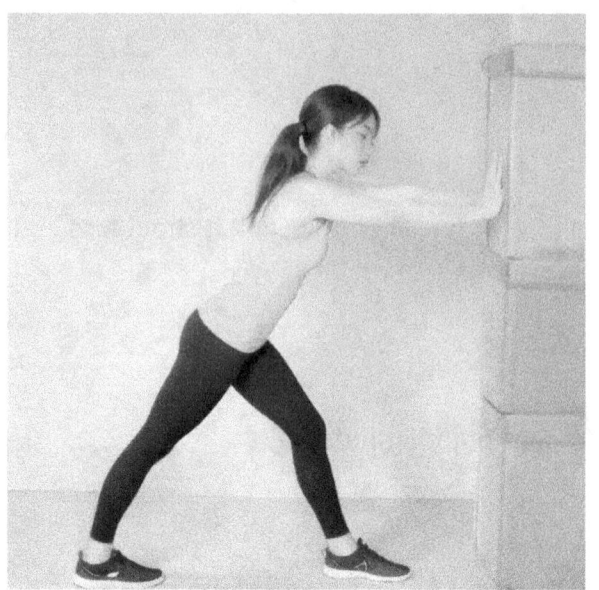 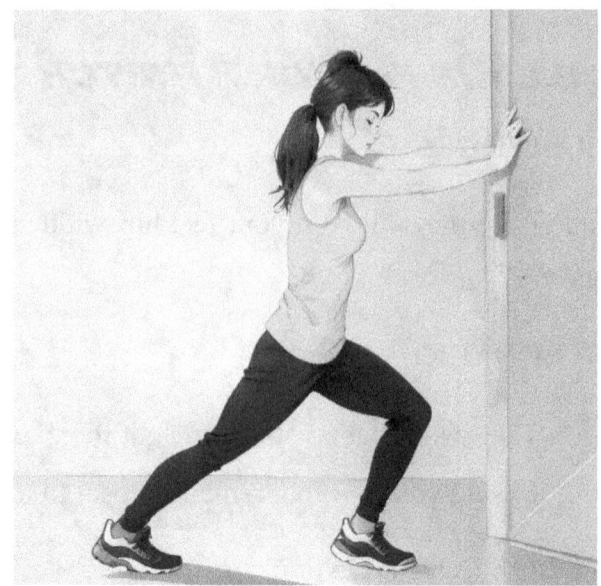

8. MODIFICATIONS:

- If you need a deeper stretch, you can raise your arms overhead while maintaining contact with the wall.
- Experiment with the distance between your feet to find the most comfortable stretch.

9. FREQUENCY:

- Incorporate this stretch into your warm-up routine or after a workout.
- Perform 2-3 sets on each leg to enhance flexibility.

10. CAUTION:

- Avoid pushing into sharp pain; the stretch should be comfortable and controlled.
- If you have any pre-existing hip issues, consult with a healthcare professional before attempting this stretch.

Add the Wall Hip Flexor Stretch to your routine to alleviate tightness and enhance the flexibility of your hip flexors. This stretch is particularly beneficial for individuals with sedentary lifestyles or those who engage in activities that involve prolonged sitting.

WALL QUAD STRETCH

1. SETUP:

- Stand facing the wall with your feet hip-width apart.
- Place one hand on the wall for support, ensuring your arm is straight.

2. LIFTING THE FOOT:

- Bend your right knee and lift your right foot towards your buttocks.
- Reach back with your right hand and grab your ankle or the top of your foot.

3. ALIGNMENT:

- Ensure that your standing leg is slightly bent to maintain stability.
- Keep your knees close together, avoiding any outward splaying.

4. POSTURE:

- Stand tall, engaging your core for stability.
- Maintain a neutral spine without arching your back excessively.

5. STRETCHING:

Gently pull your right foot towards your buttocks until you feel a comfortable stretch in the front of your right thigh (quadriceps).

6. BREATHING:

Inhale as you lift your foot towards your buttocks. Exhale as you deepen the stretch.

7. HOLDING THE STRETCH:

Hold the stretch for 15-30 seconds, feeling the tension release in your quadriceps. Focus on relaxing into the stretch rather than forcing it.

8. SWITCHING SIDES:

Release the right foot and switch to the left side, following the same steps.

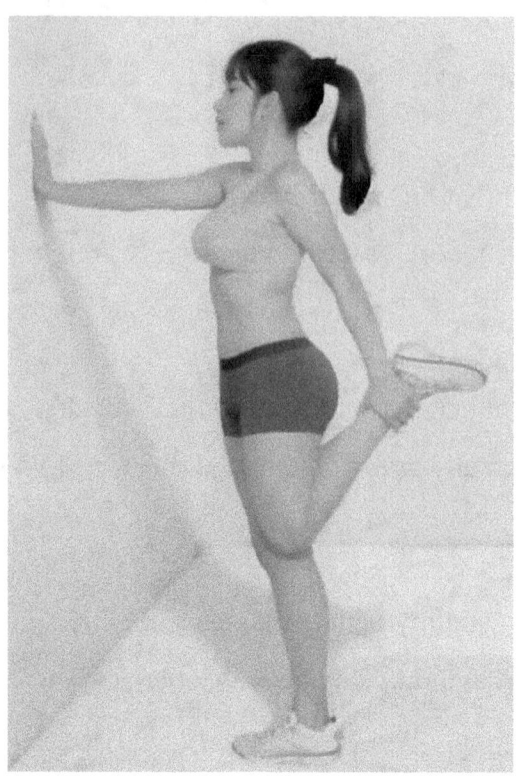

9. COMMON MISTAKES TO AVOID:

- Avoid excessive arching of the lower back; maintain a neutral spine.
- Ensure a controlled and gradual lift of the foot to prevent overstretching.

10. BENEFITS:

- Improves flexibility in the quadriceps.
- Alleviates tension in the front of the thighs.
- Enhances overall lower body mobility.

11. INCORPORATION INTO YOUR ROUTINE:

- Include the Wall Quad Stretch in your warm-up or cool-down routine.
- Perform after a workout to release tension in the quadriceps.

Adding the Wall Quad Stretch to your routine contributes to improved flexibility and reduced muscle tension, promoting overall lower body well-being. Enjoy the benefits of this simple yet effective stretch for enhanced mobility.

BALANCE

SINGLE LEG STANCE

1. SETUP:

Begin by standing with your feet hip-width apart and your weight evenly distributed.

2. FOCUS AND ALIGNMENT:

Choose a focal point in front of you to maintain balance. Engage your core muscles to stabilize your spine.

3. SHIFT YOUR WEIGHT:

Shift your weight onto one leg while lifting the other foot slightly off the ground. Find a comfortable position for your lifted foot, either by keeping the toes lightly touching the ground or placing the sole against the inner calf.

4. MAINTAIN BALANCE:

- Keep your standing knee slightly bent to maintain stability.
- Use your arms for balance by extending them to the sides or placing your hands on your hips.

5. GAZE AND BREATHING:

- Fix your gaze on the chosen focal point to help with balance.
- Breathe steadily and maintain a relaxed posture throughout the exercise.

6. HOLDING THE STANCE:

- Aim to hold the single-leg stance for 20-30 seconds initially.
- As you gain strength and stability, gradually increase the duration.

7. SWITCHING LEGS:

- Lower the lifted foot back to the ground.
- Shift your weight to the opposite leg and repeat the exercise on the other side.

8. PROGRESSIVE CHALLENGES:

- To intensify the exercise, try closing your eyes while maintaining the single-leg stance.
- Increase the duration gradually to challenge your balance further.

9. COMMON MISTAKES TO AVOID:

- Avoid locking your standing knee; keep it slightly bent.
- Ensure that your hips remain level and don't tilt to one side.
- Maintain proper alignment to prevent unnecessary strain on your joints.

10. BENEFITS:

- Enhances balance and proprioception.
- Strengthens stabilizing muscles in the legs and core.
- Improves focus and concentration.

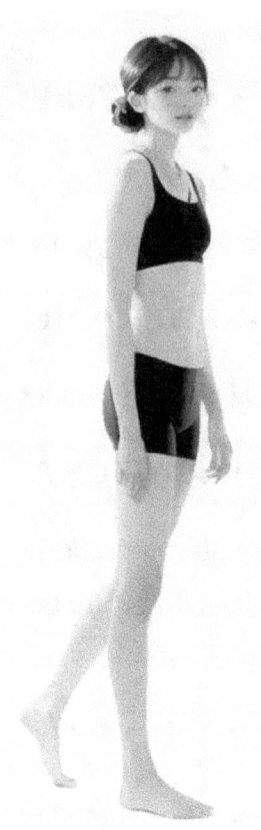

SINGLE LEG WALL STAND

1. SETUP:

- Begin by standing with your back against the wall and feet hip-width apart.
- Engage your core for stability and ensure a straight alignment from head to heels.

2. SHIFTING WEIGHT:

- Shift your weight onto one leg while lifting the opposite foot off the ground.
- Place the sole of the lifted foot against the wall, finding a comfortable height.

3. POSTURE AND ALIGNMENT:

- Keep your standing knee slightly bent for stability.

- Maintain a neutral spine with shoulders relaxed.
- Extend your arms forward or place them on your hips for balance.

4. FOCUS ON STABILITY:

Concentrate on stabilizing through the standing leg and engaging the muscles in your core and hip. Find a focal point to help with balance and focus your gaze.

5. HOLDING THE POSITION:

- Hold the single-leg wall stand for the desired duration, starting with 15-30 seconds and progressing as you build strength.
- Breathe steadily and maintain control throughout the exercise.

6. ALTERNATING LEGS:

- After completing the hold on one leg, gently lower the lifted foot to the ground.
- Shift your weight to the other leg and repeat the single-leg wall stand on the opposite side.

7. BREATHING:

- Inhale as you lift your foot and shift your weight.
- Exhale and maintain a steady breath during the hold.

8. COMMON MISTAKES TO AVOID:

Avoid locking the standing knee; keep a slight bend to prevent strain. Ensure the lifted foot is placed against the wall at a comfortable height to avoid overextension.

9. BENEFITS:

- Improves balance and proprioception.
- Strengthens the muscles in the standing leg, particularly the hip and thigh.
- Enhances overall stability and control.

10. INCORPORATION INTO YOUR ROUTINE:

- Include the single-leg wall stand as part of your warm-up or balance training routine.
- Gradually increase the duration as your balance improves.

Adding the single-leg wall stand to your repertoire not only enhances your balance but also strengthens key lower body muscles. Enjoy the sense of stability and control as you progress in this exercise.

WALL LEG SWING

1. SETUP:

- Find an open space with a clear wall in front of you.
- Stand facing the wall, with your feet hip-width apart.
- Place your hands on the wall for support, ensuring they are at shoulder height.

2. INITIATE THE SWING:

- Lift one leg off the ground, bending the knee slightly.
- Swing the leg forward and backward in a controlled manner.
- Keep your standing leg slightly bent to maintain balance.

3. SIDE-TO-SIDE MOTION:

- After a few swings in the forward and backward direction, switch to a side-to-side motion.
- Swing your leg from side to side while maintaining stability.

4. ADJUST YOUR RANGE:

- Control the height and range of your leg swings based on your flexibility and comfort.
- Gradually increase the height and intensity as your muscles warm up.

5. ENGAGE YOUR CORE:

- Keep your core muscles engaged to stabilize your body.
- Focus on maintaining good posture throughout the exercise.

6. BREATHING:

Inhale as you swing your leg forward or to the side. Exhale as you bring your leg back to the starting position.

7. SWITCH LEGS:

After completing the recommended number of swings with one leg, switch to the other. Ensure both legs receive equal attention during the exercise.

8. COMMON MISTAKES TO AVOID:

- Avoid overly forceful swings; maintain control to prevent strain.
- Keep your standing knee slightly bent to protect your joints.
- Do not lock your standing knee during the exercise.

9. BENEFITS:

- Improves hip flexibility and mobility.
- Activates and warms up the muscles in your legs.
- Enhances balance and coordination.

10. INCORPORATION INTO YOUR ROUTINE:

Consider incorporating this exercise into a dynamic stretching routine for overall flexibility.

Wall Leg Swings provide a dynamic and effective way to warm up your lower body, enhance flexibility, and activate key muscles. Incorporate this exercise into your fitness routine to promote improved leg mobility and balance.

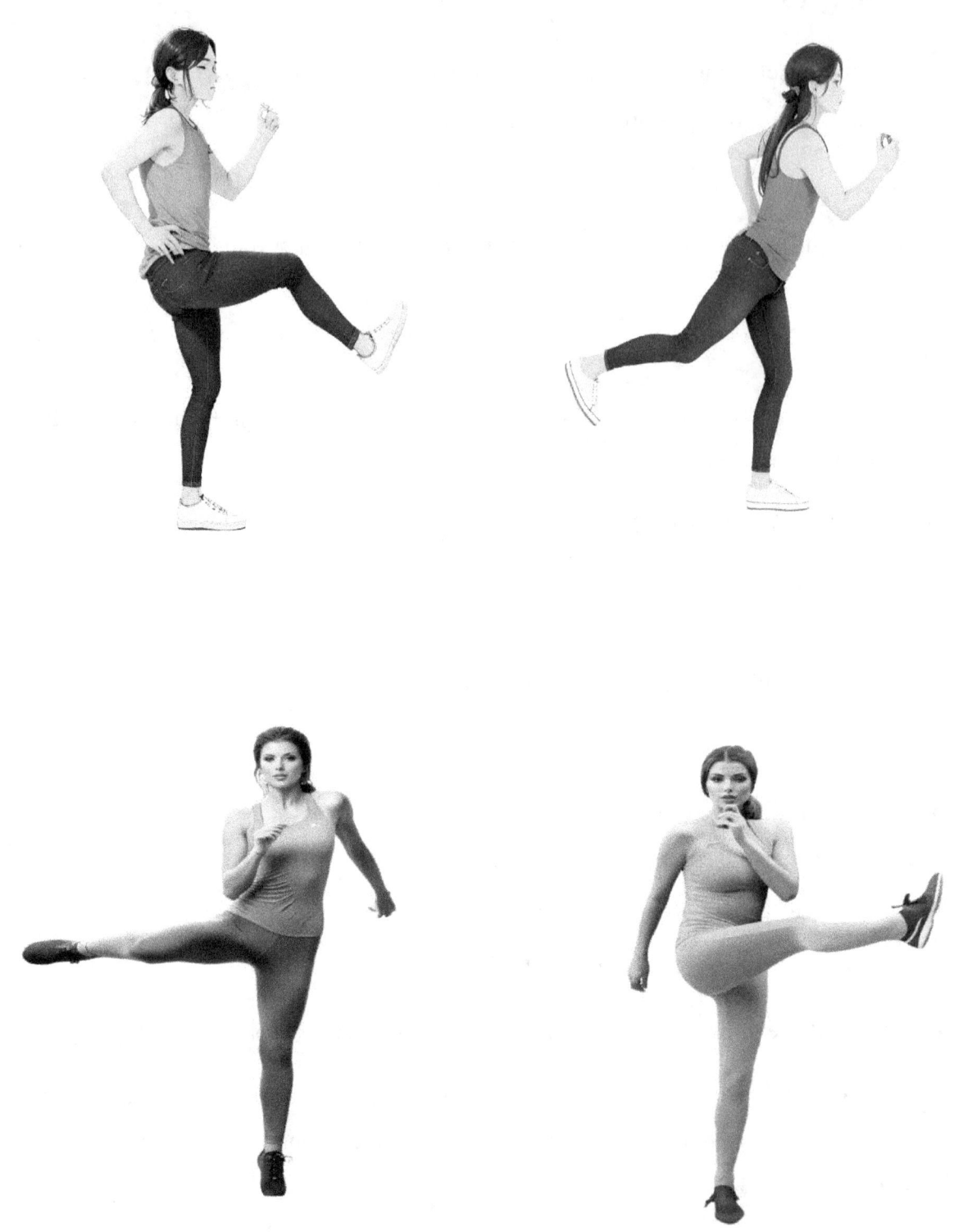

WALL HEEL-TO-TOE WALK

1. STARTING POSITION:

Stand facing the wall with your feet hip-width apart. Place your hands lightly on the wall for support.

2. INITIATE THE MOVEMENT:

- Lift your right heel off the ground, keeping your toes in contact with the floor.
- Begin walking forward by placing the heel of your right foot directly in front of the toes of your left foot.
- Maintain a straight line as you move, placing one foot directly in front of the other.

3. HEEL-TO-TOE CONTACT:

Each time you take a step, ensure that your heel touches the floor first, followed by the toes of the opposite foot. This creates a seamless heel-to-toe walking pattern.

4. SLOW AND CONTROLLED MOVEMENT:

- Perform the heel-to-toe walk in a slow and controlled manner.
- Focus on balance and coordination throughout the exercise.

5. USE WALL SUPPORT WHEN NEEDED:

If you feel unsteady, utilize the wall for support by keeping your hands lightly in contact with it.

Gradually decrease reliance on the wall as your balance improves.

6. STRAIGHT POSTURE:

- Maintain an upright posture throughout the exercise, engaging your core muscles.
- Keep your gaze forward to assist with balance.

7. ALTERNATE LEG MOVEMENT:

- Continue the heel-to-toe walking pattern, alternating between the right and left legs.
- Strive for a smooth and fluid motion.

8. BREATHING:

Breathe naturally throughout the exercise, avoiding shallow breaths. Inhale and exhale in a relaxed manner.

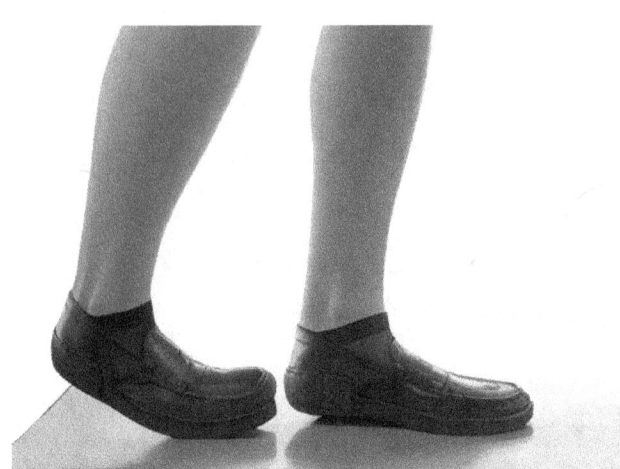 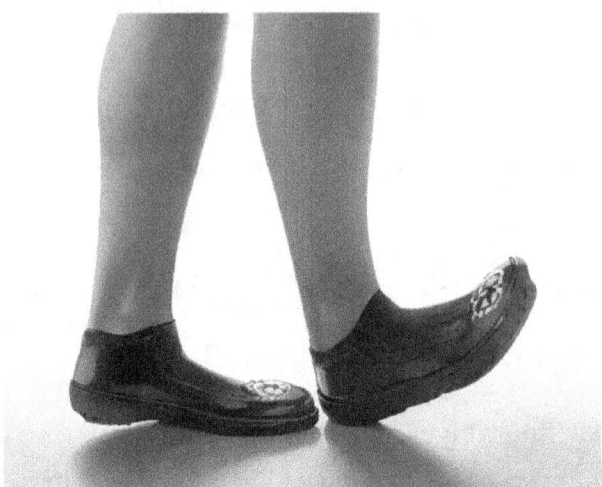

9. REPETITIONS AND SETS:

Perform the wall heel-to-toe walk for a designated distance or time. Start with a few repetitions and gradually increase as your balance improves.

10. BENEFITS:

- Enhances balance and coordination.
- Strengthens the muscles of the lower body.
- Improves proprioception (awareness of body position).

Incorporate the wall heel-to-toe walk into your routine to enhance balance, stability, and overall lower body strength. This simple yet effective exercise can be adapted to various fitness levels and provides a valuable foundation for improving your sense of balance.

WALL BALANCE KNEE RAISES

1. INITIAL SETUP:

Stand with your back against the wall, ensuring your feet are hip-width apart. Maintain a straight posture with your shoulders relaxed and core engaged.

2. HAND PLACEMENT:

Place your hands lightly on the wall for support.

3. LIFTING THE KNEE:

- Begin by lifting one knee towards your chest, engaging your abdominal muscles.
- Focus on maintaining your balance as you lift the knee as high as comfortably possible.

4. CONTROLLED MOVEMENT:

- Avoid any sudden or jerky movements; perform the knee raise in a controlled manner.
- Feel the activation in your lower abdominal muscles as you lift the knee.

5. HOLDING THE POSITION:

- Once the knee is raised, hold the position for a brief moment, maintaining your balance.
- Keep your standing leg slightly bent to enhance stability.

6. LOWERING THE KNEE:

Gradually lower the raised knee back to the starting position. Control the descent to engage the muscles throughout the entire movement.

7. ALTERNATE LEGS:

- Repeat the exercise with the opposite leg.
- Aim for a smooth and coordinated movement with each repetition.

8. BREATHING:

Inhale as you lift the knee. Exhale as you lower the knee back to the starting position.

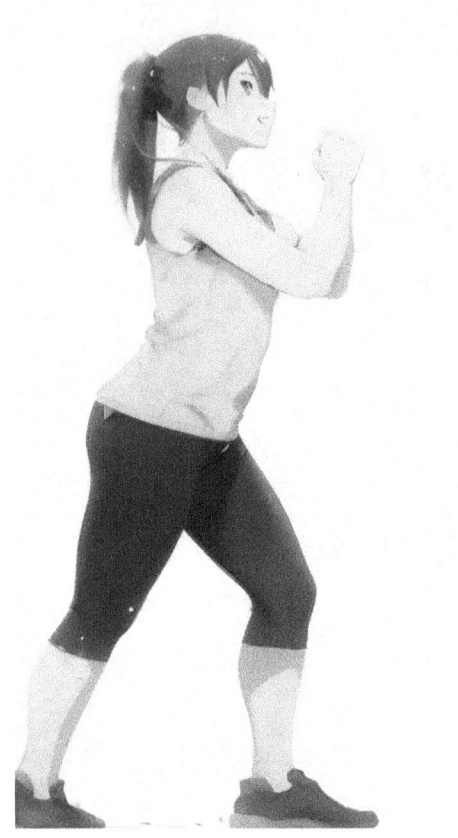 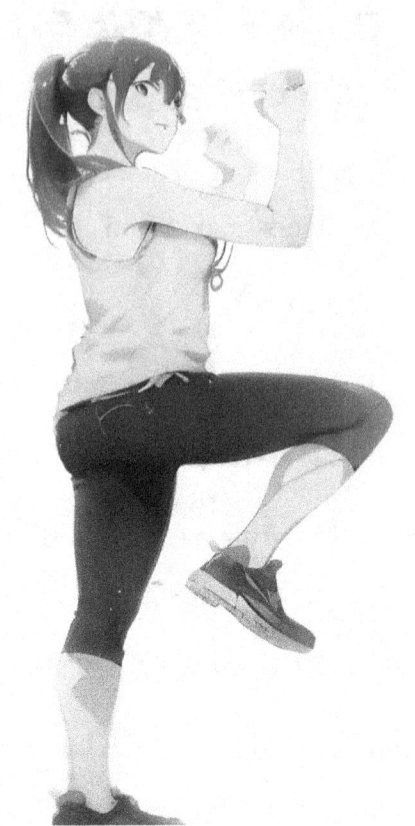

9. COMMON MISTAKES TO AVOID:

- Avoid leaning too heavily on the wall; use it for support without relying on it entirely.
- Ensure that the raised knee is lifted towards the chest, not out to the side.

10. BENEFITS:

- Strengthens the core muscles, especially the lower abdominals.
- Enhances balance and stability.
- Improves hip flexor flexibility.

Include Wall Balance Knee Raises as part of your warm-up or as a standalone exercise for core activation and balance enhancement.

Gradually increase the number of repetitions as your strength and balance improve.

CHAPTER 9 - FUN PARTNER WORKOUTS

ENGAGING EXERCISES THAT CAN BE DONE WITH A FRIEND FOR ADDED MOTIVATION

Enhance your fitness journey by adding a social and motivational element. These partner workouts are designed to make exercising enjoyable, foster camaraderie, and keep you motivated. Grab a friend, and let the fun begin with these engaging exercises.

WALL PILATES BALL PASS

1. SETUP:

- Stand facing your partner, maintaining a comfortable distance between you.
- Both partners should have a Pilates ball in hand.

2. STARTING POSITION:

Begin in a standing position with your feet hip-width apart. Hold the Pilates ball with both hands, extending your arms forward.

3. PASSING THE BALL:

- Simultaneously, both partners pass the Pilates ball to each other.
- Focus on coordination and timing to smoothly transfer the ball.
- Engage your core throughout the movement to stabilize your body.

4. CHALLENGE YOUR CORE:

- Lift one leg off the ground during the ball pass to increase the engagement of your core muscles.
- Alternate legs to maintain balance and target different muscle groups.

5. TIMING AND RHYTHM:

- Coordinate with your partner to establish a steady and rhythmic pace.
- Aim for a seamless flow of ball passes, maintaining control over the movement.

6. ENCOURAGEMENT AND COMMUNICATION:

Encourage each other throughout the exercise, fostering a positive and supportive atmosphere. Communication is key to syncing movements and ensuring a successful workout.

7. REPETITIONS AND SETS:

- Begin with a moderate number of repetitions and sets, gradually increasing as you build strength and coordination.
- Pay attention to your partner's comfort level and adjust intensity accordingly.

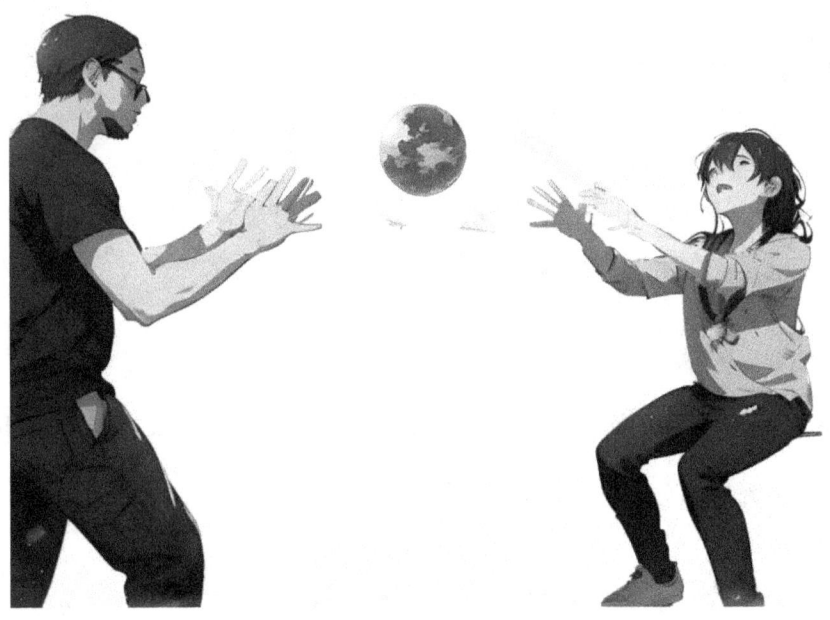

8. VARIATIONS:

Experiment with different passing patterns, such as diagonal passes or overhead passes, to keep the exercise interesting. Modify the distance between partners based on skill level and space availability.

9. COOLDOWN:

Conclude the Wall Pilates Ball Pass with a gentle cool-down, incorporating stretches for the shoulders, core, and arms.

BENEFITS:

- Strengthens the core muscles, including abdominals and obliques.

- Enhances coordination and teamwork skills.

- Adds an element of fun and engagement to your Pilates routine.

PARTNER WALL SQUATS

1. SETUP:

- Stand back-to-back with your partner, ensuring your spines are aligned.

- Maintain a hip-width distance between your feet.

- Both partners should have their feet planted firmly on the ground.

2. SYNCHRONIZED MOVEMENT:

- Simultaneously lower your bodies into a squat position by bending your knees.

- Aim to create a 90-degree angle with your knees, keeping your backs against each other.

- Maintain a neutral spine throughout the movement.

3. TEAMWORK AND SUPPORT:

- Lean into each other's backs for added stability and support.

- Ensure both partners maintain proper form by aligning their knees over their ankles.

- Use each other's presence to deepen the squat without compromising form.

4. FULL RANGE OF MOTION:

- Lower your bodies as far as comfortable, aiming for a full range of motion.

- Focus on engaging your quadriceps, hamstrings, and glutes during the descent.

- Keep your core activated for added stability.

5. UPWARD MOVEMENT:

- Push through your heels to return to the starting position.

- Straighten your legs fully, ensuring both partners rise together.
- Maintain a controlled pace throughout the movement.

6. REPETITIONS:

Perform the desired number of repetitions, communicating with your partner to synchronize your movements. Start with a manageable number of reps and gradually increase as your strength improves.

7. BREATHING:

Inhale as you descend into the squat. Exhale as you push through your heels to return to the starting position.

8. COMMON MISTAKES TO AVOID:

Ensure your knees do not go beyond your toes to prevent strain. Keep your back straight and avoid rounding your shoulders.

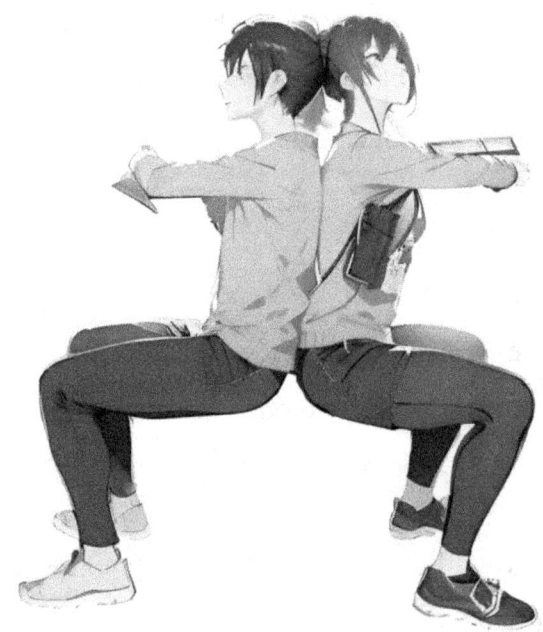

9. TEAM ENCOURAGEMENT:

- Motivate each other throughout the exercise with words of encouragement.
- Celebrate your joint effort and progress.

Partner wall squats provide a unique and enjoyable way to challenge your lower body while building a sense of teamwork. Incorporate this exercise into your routine for a fun and effective workout experience with a fitness companion.

WALL PLANK HIGH FIVES

1. SETUP:

- Begin by facing your partner in a plank position, ensuring that you are a comfortable distance apart.
- Place your hands directly beneath your shoulders, and maintain a strong, straight line from head to heels.

2. COORDINATED MOVEMENT:

- Lift your right hand off the ground and reach towards your partner for a high five.
- Simultaneously, your partner does the same with their right hand.
- Focus on maintaining a stable plank position throughout the movement.

3. EXECUTION:

- Execute the high five with your partner, making contact in the air between your two hands.
- Keep your core engaged and hips level to ensure stability.
- Lower your right hand back to the ground, returning to the plank position.

4. ALTERNATE HANDS:

Repeat the movement, but this time, lift your left hand for the high five while your partner does the same.

Continue alternating hands for the duration of the exercise.

5. BREATHING:

Inhale as you prepare to lift your hand for the high five. Exhale as you execute the high five and lower your hand back to the ground.

6. COMMUNICATION:

- Maintain clear communication with your partner to synchronize the high-fiving motion.
- Encourage each other throughout the exercise to stay motivated.

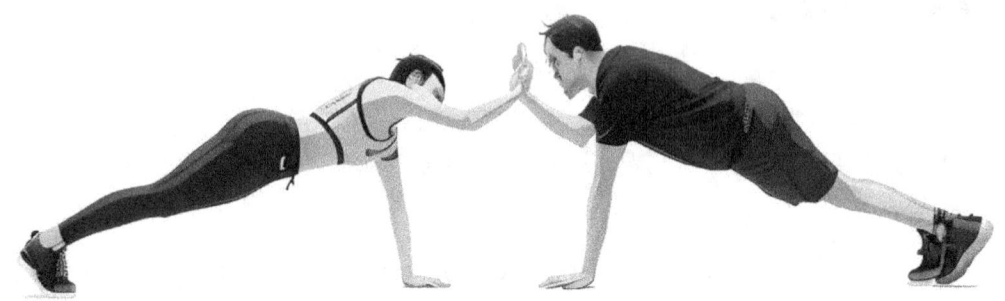

7. COMMON MISTAKES TO AVOID:

Avoid letting your hips sag or rise during the high-five motion; keep a straight line from head to heels.

Ensure both partners are equally participating in the movement for balanced engagement.

8. BENEFITS:

Enhances core stability and strength.

Promotes coordination between partners.

Adds a fun and interactive element to plank exercises.

9. INCORPORATION INTO YOUR ROUTINE:

Include Wall Plank High Fives as a dynamic and engaging component of your partner workout routine.

Aim for smooth and controlled movements, emphasizing proper form and coordination.

WALL SEATED TWIST PARTNER STRETCH

1. SETUP:

Sit up tall, lengthening your spine, and ensure a comfortable seated position.

3. INITIATE THE TWIST:

They both inhale. You both turn to your right sides as you release the breath. Using your right hand, reach back and seize your partner's left knee. Execute this at the same time. Your own right knees will be grasped by the left hands.

Keep your posture straight and tall, and try to twist a little bit further with each exhalation. Your partner will help you by doing the twist as well! Try to get both of you as close to the floor as you can; this will keep you grounded and prevent you from falling. If you lean too close to each other, one of you will fall to the ground.

4. HOLD THE STRETCH:

- Hold the twist for 15-30 seconds, allowing your muscles to relax and elongate.
- Communicate with your partner to ensure both are comfortable with the stretch intensity.

5. REPEAT ON THE OPPOSITE SIDE:

- Slowly return to the center position and then initiate the twist in the opposite direction.
- Feel the stretch on the other side of your torso, promoting flexibility and mobility.

6. BREATHING TECHNIQUE:

Inhale deeply through your nose as you sit tall. Exhale slowly as you deepen the twist, encouraging relaxation.

7. COMMUNICATION IS KEY:

Maintain open communication with your partner during the stretch. Adjust the intensity based on both partners' comfort levels.

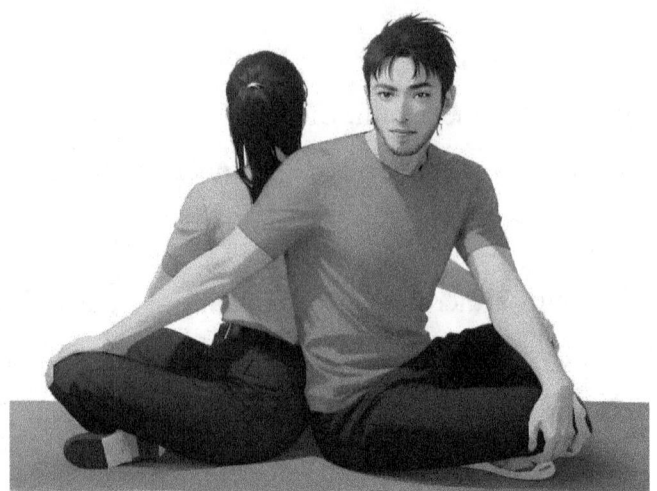 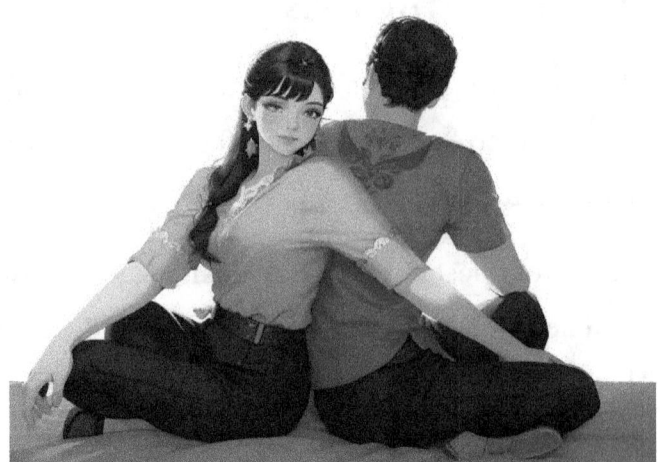

8. BENEFITS:

Increases flexibility in the spine and torso.

Promotes a gentle stretch in the obliques and lower back.

Enhances joint mobility in the hips.

9. CAUTION:

Avoid forcing the stretch; it should be comfortable and gentle.

If you experience any discomfort, communicate with your partner and adjust as needed.

10. INCORPORATION INTO YOUR ROUTINE:

Include the Wall Seated Twist Partner Stretch as part of your cool-down or flexibility routine.

Enjoy the shared experience with your partner, fostering a sense of connection.

Partner stretches like the Wall Seated Twist add a playful and enjoyable element to your fitness journey while promoting flexibility and joint health.

CHAPTER 10 - 28-DAY CHALLENGE TO TRANSFORM YOUR BODY

Welcome to the transformative 28-day Wall Pilates Challenge, a journey crafted to reshape your body, empower your mind, and elevate your overall well-being. This comprehensive program is designed for individuals of all fitness levels, guiding you through a strategic progression of exercises that target different muscle groups, enhance flexibility, and foster a deeper mind-body connection.

WEEK 1: CORE SCULPT & STRENGTHEN

DAY 1: FOUNDATION DAY

Wall Mountain Climbers

Isometric Wall Plank Hold

Wall Leg Raises

DAY 2: CORE ACTIVATION

Wall Dead Bug

Wall Dead Bug with Arm Slide

High Wall Knee Tucks (Inverted)

DAY 3: CORE CHALLENGE

Vertical Wall Sit & Twist

Wall Oblique Crunches

DAY 4: RECOVERY AND STRETCH

Wall Forward Fold

Wall Chest Opener

Wall Tricep Stretch

DAY 5: FULL CORE ENGAGEMENT

Repeat Day 1 exercises

DAY 6: FLEXIBILITY FOCUS

Wall Hip Flexor Stretch

Wall Quad Stretch

DAY 7:

Rest and Recovery

WEEK 2: UPPER BODY TONE & DEFINE

DAY 8: UPPER BODY FOUNDATION

Wall Row

Wall Row Isohold

Hinge to Wall

DAY 9: TRICEPS AND CHEST

Wall Tricep Extension

Wall ER

Wall Push-Up Plus

DAY 10: PUSH AND PULL

Wall Push Up

Floor Push Up

DAY 11: RECOVERY AND STRETCH

Wall Forward Fold

Wall Chest Opener

Wall Tricep Stretch

DAY 12: UPPER BODY ENDURANCE

Repeat Day 8 exercises

DAY 13: FLEXIBILITY FOCUS

Wall Hip Flexor Stretch

Wall Triceps Stretch

DAY 14:

Rest and Recovery

WEEK 3: LOWER BODY SHAPE & DEFINE

DAY 15: LOWER BODY FOUNDATION

Wall Squat Holds

Elevated Wall Lunges

Wall-Supported Pistol Squats

DAY 16: GLUTES ACTIVATION

Glute Bridge Wall Slides

Wall Side Leg Lifts

DAY 17: SQUATS AND PULSES

Wall Squat with Calf Raise

Elevated Stallion Pulses

DAY 18: RECOVERY AND STRETCH

Wall Forward Fold

Wall Chest Opener

Wall Quad Stretch

DAY 19: FULL LOWER BODY CHALLENGE

Repeat Day 15 exercises

DAY 20: FLEXIBILITY FOCUS

Wall Hip Flexor Stretch

Wall Quad Stretch

DAY 21:

Rest and Recovery

WEEK 4: BALANCE AND FLEXIBILITY

DAY 22: FULL BODY BALANCE

Single Leg Stance

Single Leg Wall Stand

Wall Leg Swing

DAY 23: WALKING AND BALANCE

Wall Heel-to-Toe Walk

Wall Balance Knee Raises

DAY 24: FLEXIBILITY AND BALANCE

Wall- Assisted Leg Extension

Wall Cossack Squat

DAY 25: RECOVERY AND STRETCH

Wall Forward Fold

Wall Chest Opener

Wall Tricep Stretch

DAY 26: CORE AND BALANCE INTEGRATION

High Wall Glute Kickbacks

Wall-Facing Squat

DAY 27: FULL BODY CHALLENGE

Repeat exercises from Days 22-26

DAY 28:

Celebration and Reflection

Rest and Reflect on Achievements

Remember to maintain proper form, listen to your body, and adjust the intensity as needed. Enjoy your 28-day journey to a transformed and stronger you!

CHAPTER 11 - BONUS CONTENT

FUEL YOUR FITNESS: ENERGIZING SMOOTHIES & BALANCED MEALS.

In your journey to transform your body through Wall Pilates, nutrition plays a crucial role. Fueling your body with the right nutrients enhances your energy levels, supports muscle recovery, and accelerates your overall fitness progress. Here's a guide to creating energizing smoothies and balanced meals that complement your Wall Pilates workouts.

ENERGIZING SMOOTHIE RECIPES:

CITRUS BOOST SMOOTHIE:

Ingredients:

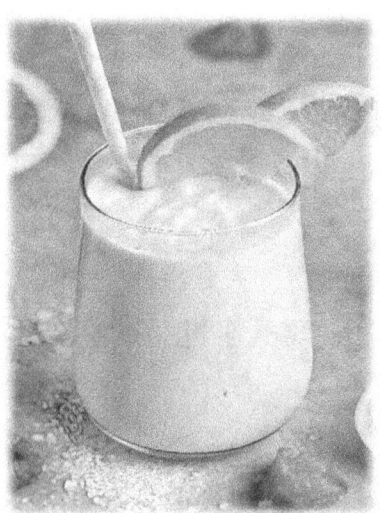

- 1 orange, peeled and segmented
- 1/2 grapefruit, peeled and segmented
- 1 banana
- 1/2 cup Greek yogurt
- Ice cubes

Preparation:

- Place all ingredients in a blender.
- Blend until smooth.
- Pour into a glass and enjoy the refreshing boost!

Benefits:

- Rich in vitamin C for immune support.
- Provides a burst of natural energy.

BERRY BLAST ANTIOXIDANT SMOOTHIE:

Ingredients:

- 1 cup mixed berries (strawberries, blueberries, raspberries)
- Handful of spinach leaves
- 1 cup almond milk
- 1 tablespoon chia seeds

Preparation:

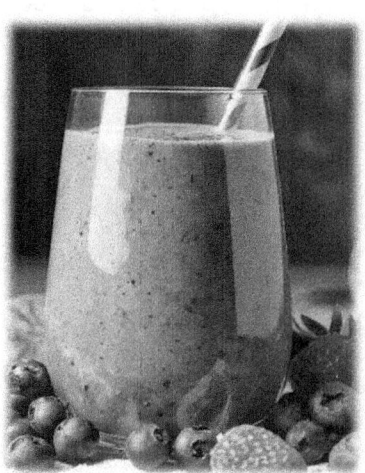

- Combine all ingredients in a blender.
- Blend until smooth.
- Pour into a glass and savor the antioxidant-rich goodness.

Benefits:

- High in antioxidants for cellular health.
- Spinach adds iron and vitamins.

PINEAPPLE MINT DELIGHT:

Ingredients:

- 1 cup pineapple chunks
- Handful of mint leaves
- 1/2 cup coconut water
- 1/2 cup yogurt

Preparation:

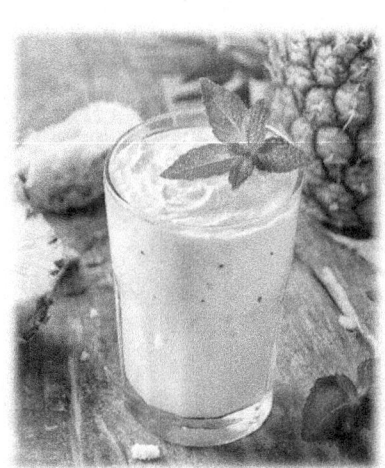

- Blend pineapple, mint, coconut water, and yogurt.
- Blend until smooth.
- Pour into a glass, and enjoy the tropical delight.

Benefits:

- Pineapple provides digestive enzymes.
- Mint aids digestion and adds a refreshing flavor.

MANGO TURMERIC ELIXIR:

Ingredients:

- 1 ripe mango, peeled and diced
- 1/2 teaspoon turmeric
- 1/2 cup Greek yogurt
- 1 cup almond milk

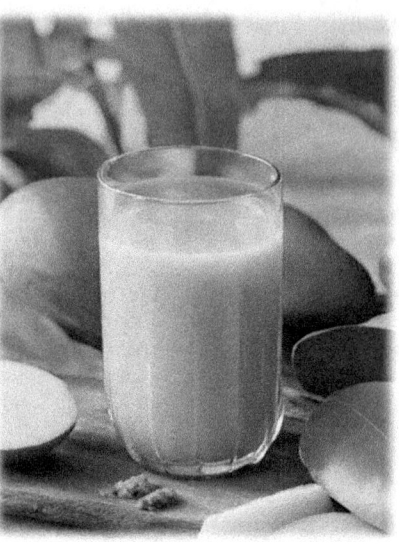

Preparation:

- Combine mango, turmeric, Greek yogurt, and almond milk in a blender.
- Blend until creamy and smooth.
- Pour into a glass for a nourishing elixir.

Benefits:

- Turmeric provides anti-inflammatory properties.
- Mango adds natural sweetness and vitamins.

CHOCOLATE PEANUT BUTTER PROTEIN SHAKE:

Ingredients:

- 2 tablespoons cocoa powder
- 1 banana
- 2 tablespoons peanut butter
- 1 scoop protein powder
- 1 cup milk

Preparation:

- Blend cocoa powder, banana, peanut butter, protein powder, and milk.
- Blend until well combined.
- Pour into a glass for a protein-packed treat.

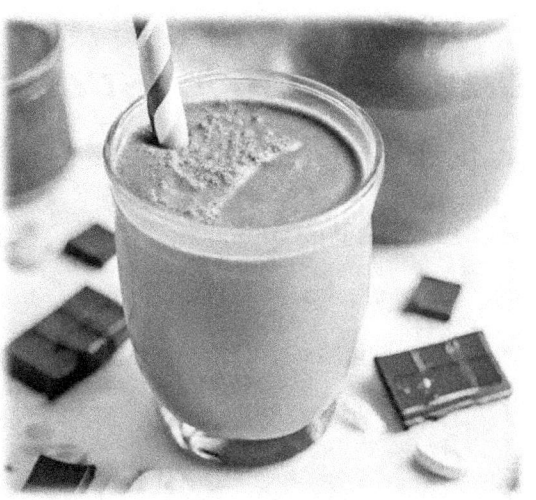

Benefits:

- High protein content for muscle recovery.
- Cocoa and banana provide a delightful flavor.

GREEN TEA & BERRY FUSION:

Ingredients:

- 1 cup brewed green tea, cooled
- 1 cup mixed berries
- 1 tablespoon honey
- 1/2 cup Greek yogurt

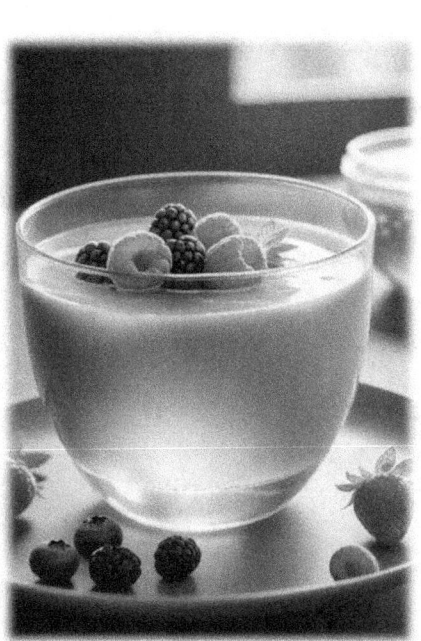

Preparation:

- Combine green tea, mixed berries, honey, and Greek yogurt in a blender.
- Blend until smooth.
- Pour into a glass and enjoy the refreshing fusion.

Benefits:

- Green tea offers antioxidants and a gentle caffeine boost.
- Berries contribute vitamins and fiber.

BALANCED MEAL IDEAS:

QUINOA CHICKPEA BUDDHA BOWL:

Ingredients:

- 1 cup cooked quinoa
- 1 cup chickpeas, roasted
- Assorted roasted vegetables
- Tahini dressing

Preparation:

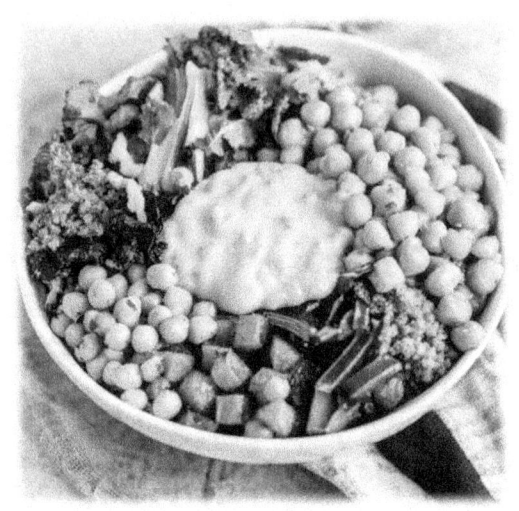

- Arrange quinoa, chickpeas, and roasted vegetables in a bowl.
- Drizzle with tahini dressing.
- Toss and enjoy this nourishing Buddha bowl.

Benefits:

- Quinoa provides a complete protein source.
- Chickpeas offer fiber and plant-based protein.

SALMON AVOCADO QUINOA SALAD:

Ingredients:

- Grilled salmon fillet
- 1 cup cooked quinoa
- Sliced avocado
- Cherry tomatoes

Preparation:

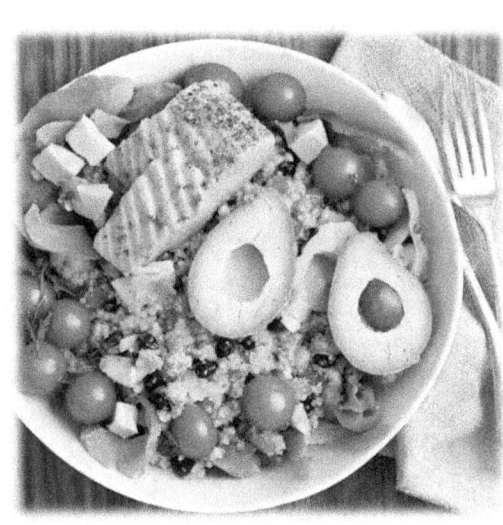

- Place quinoa in a bowl, top with grilled salmon, avocado, and cherry tomatoes.
- Season to taste.

Benefits:

- Salmon provides omega-3 fatty acids for heart health.
- Avocado adds healthy fats and creamy texture.

MEDITERRANEAN LENTIL SOUP:

Ingredients:

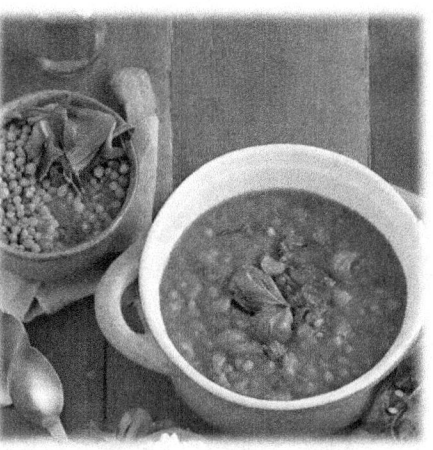

- 1 cup lentils
- Tomatoes, spinach, feta
- Olive oil

Preparation:

- Cook lentils according to package instructions.
- Add tomatoes, spinach, and crumbled feta.
- Drizzle with olive oil and savor this Mediterranean-inspired soup.

Benefits:

- Lentils offer a rich source of plant-based protein.
- Spinach provides iron and vitamins.

STIR-FRIED TOFU & VEGETABLE QUINOA:

Ingredients:

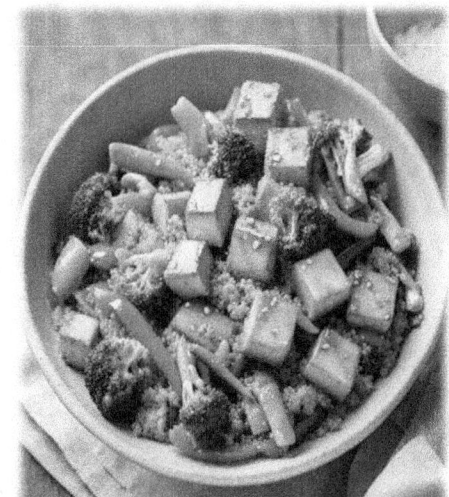

- Tofu cubes
- Mixed vegetables (broccoli, bell peppers, snap peas)
- Quinoa
- Soy sauce

Preparation:

- Stir-fry tofu and mixed vegetables.
- Serve over cooked quinoa.
- Drizzle with soy sauce and enjoy this flavorful stir-fry.

Benefits:

- Tofu contributes plant-based protein.
- Colorful vegetables offer a variety of nutrients.

CHICKEN & AVOCADO WRAP:

Ingredients:

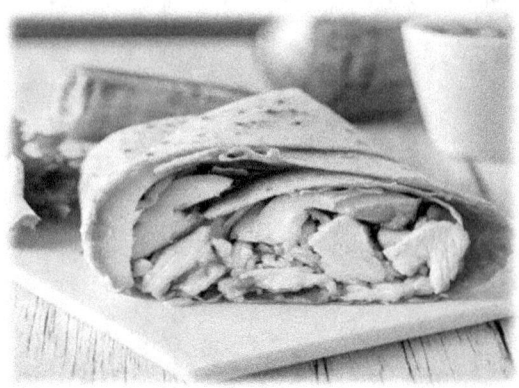

- Grilled chicken slices
- Avocado
- Lettuce
- Whole-grain wrap

Preparation:

- Lay out the wrap, add chicken, lettuce, and avocado slices.
- Wrap it up for a quick and tasty chicken avocado wrap.

Benefits:

- Chicken provides lean protein.
- Avocado adds healthy fats and creaminess.

SWEET POTATO BLACK BEAN CHILI:

Ingredients:

- Diced sweet potatoes
- Black beans
- Tomatoes, chili spices

Preparation:

- Combine all the ingredients and simmer until flavors meld into a comforting chili.

Benefits:

- Sweet potatoes offer complex carbohydrates and fiber; Black beans provide plant-based protein and fiber.

TRAIL MIX CRUNCH:

Ingredients:

Almonds, cashews, dried cranberries, dark chocolate chips

Preparation:

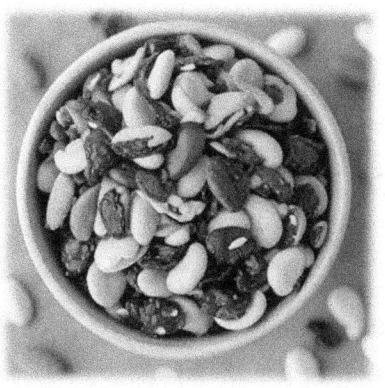

- Mix almonds, cashews, dried cranberries, and dark chocolate chips.
- Grab a handful for a satisfying trail mix crunch.

Benefits:

- Nuts offer healthy fats and protein.
- Dark chocolate adds antioxidants.

CAPRESE SKEWERS:

Ingredients:

Cherry tomatoes, mozzarella balls, basil leaves

Preparation:

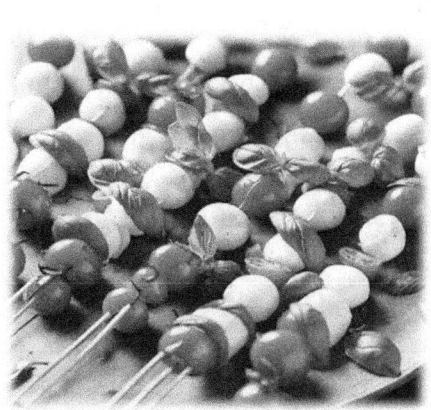

- Skewer tomatoes, mozzarella, and basil leaves.
- Drizzle with balsamic glaze for a bite-sized Caprese delight.

Benefits:

- Tomatoes provide vitamins and antioxidants.
- Mozzarella adds protein and calcium.

GREEK YOGURT & BERRY PARFAIT:

Ingredients:

Greek yogurt, granola, mixed berries, honey

Preparation:

- Layer Greek yogurt, granola, and mixed berries.
- Drizzle with honey for a parfait treat.

Benefits:

- Greek yogurt offers probiotics for gut health.
- Berries provide vitamins and antioxidants.

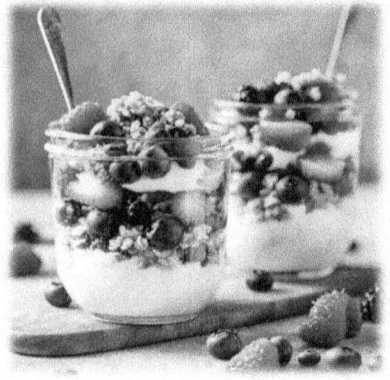

CUCUMBER HUMMUS BOATS:

Ingredients:

Cucumber slices, hummus, cherry tomatoes

Preparation:

- Fill cucumber slices with hummus.
- Top with cherry tomatoes for a refreshing hummus boat.

Benefits:

- Cucumbers hydrate and provide vitamins.
- Hummus offers plant-based protein.

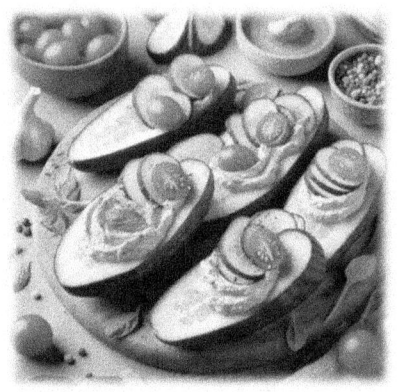

APPLE SLICES WITH ALMOND BUTTER:

Ingredients:

Apple slices, almond butter

Preparation:

- Spread almond butter on apple slices.
- Enjoy the crisp and creamy combination.

Benefits:

- Apples provide fiber and natural sweetness.
- Almond butter adds healthy fats and protein.

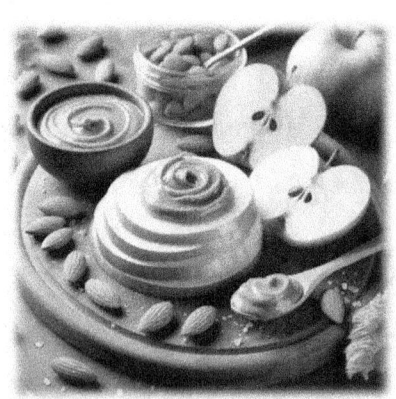

EDAMAME POWER PODS:

Ingredients:

Edamame, sea salt

Preparation:

- Steam edamame and sprinkle with sea salt.
- Pop and savor these protein-packed power pods.

Benefits:

- Edamame offers plant-based protein.
- Sea salt adds flavor without excess sodium.

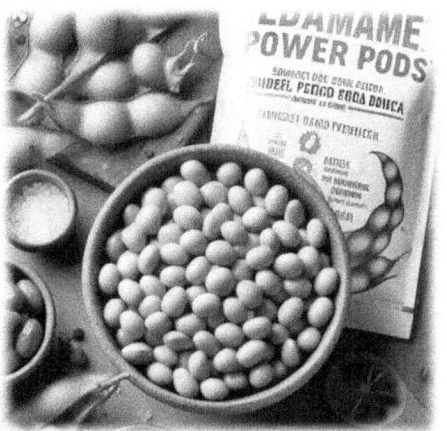

GUIDANCE ON PERSONALIZED ROUTINES & WEEKLY SCHEDULES

GUIDANCE ON PERSONALIZED ROUTINES & WEEKLY SCHEDULES:

Crafting a personalized wall Pilates routine is a dynamic process that allows you to tailor your workouts to meet your unique goals, preferences, and lifestyle. Follow this guidance to create a routine that works best for you:

1. ASSESS YOUR GOALS:

Fitness Objectives: Define what you aim to achieve—whether it's overall strength, flexibility, weight management, or targeted muscle development.

Time Commitment: Determine how much time you can realistically dedicate to Pilates each day or week.

2. IDENTIFY YOUR FITNESS LEVEL:

Beginner: If you're new to Pilates, start with foundational exercises. Gradually increase intensity as you build strength and confidence.

Intermediate: Incorporate a mix of beginner and intermediate exercises to challenge your growing abilities.

Advanced: Challenge yourself with advanced movements to maintain progression and achieve optimal results.

3. TAILOR BASED ON PREFERENCES:

Exercise Selection: Choose exercises that you enjoy and that align with your goals. A variety of movements keeps workouts interesting and engaging.

Pace: Determine whether you prefer a steady flow or more dynamic, challenging sequences.

4. DESIGNING YOUR WEEKLY SCHEDULE:

Consistency is Key: Aim for a realistic and consistent workout schedule. Consistency is crucial for progress.

Rest Days: Include rest days to allow your body to recover and prevent burnout.

Balance: Balance workouts throughout the week, incorporating a mix of core, upper body, lower body, and flexibility exercises.

5. LISTEN TO YOUR BODY:

Adapt to Your Needs: Be open to adjusting your routine based on how your body feels. If you're fatigued or sore, opt for gentler exercises.

Rest and Recovery: Allow time for rest and recovery. Adequate sleep and hydration play key roles in overall well-being.

6. GRADUAL PROGRESSION:

Incremental Challenges: Gradually increase the intensity and complexity of your workouts to challenge your body and avoid plateaus.

Reassess Regularly: Periodically reassess your fitness goals and adjust your routine accordingly.

7. MIX AND MATCH:

Variety is Key: Avoid monotony by incorporating a variety of exercises. This not only targets different muscle groups but also keeps you motivated.

Fun Workouts: Include partner workouts, wall Pilates ball exercises, or other enjoyable variations for added excitement.

8. UTILIZE GOAL SETTING TOOLS:

Goal Setting Worksheets: Use the provided goal-setting worksheets to define short-term and long-term objectives.

Progress Tracking Journal: Keep a journal to log your workouts, track achievements, and identify areas for improvement.

9. STAY ADAPTABLE:

Life Happens: Acknowledge that life may throw curveballs. Be adaptable and modify your schedule when needed without guilt.

10. SEEK PROFESSIONAL ADVICE:

Consultation: If possible, consult with a fitness professional or healthcare provider to ensure your routine aligns with your health status and goals.

PRINTABLE PROGRESS TRACKERS

WEEKLY WORKOUT PLAN

MON
FOCUS ◯ Full Body　◯ Upper Body　◯ Core　◯ Lower Body　◯ Active Rest

TUES
FOCUS ◯ Full Body　◯ Upper Body　◯ Core　◯ Lower Body　◯ Active Rest

WED
FOCUS ◯ Full Body　◯ Upper Body　◯ Core　◯ Lower Body　◯ Active Rest

THURS
FOCUS ◯ Full Body　◯ Upper Body　◯ Core　◯ Lower Body　◯ Active Rest

FRI
FOCUS ◯ Full Body　◯ Upper Body　◯ Core　◯ Lower Body　◯ Active Rest

SAT
FOCUS ◯ Full Body　◯ Upper Body　◯ Core　◯ Lower Body　◯ Active Rest

SUN
FOCUS ◯ Full Body　◯ Upper Body　◯ Core　◯ Lower Body　◯ Active Rest

WEEKLY WORKOUT PLAN

MON

FOCUS ○ Full Body ○ Upper Body ○ Core ○ Lower Body ○ Active Rest

TUES

FOCUS ○ Full Body ○ Upper Body ○ Core ○ Lower Body ○ Active Rest

WED

FOCUS ○ Full Body ○ Upper Body ○ Core ○ Lower Body ○ Active Rest

THURS

FOCUS ○ Full Body ○ Upper Body ○ Core ○ Lower Body ○ Active Rest

FRI

FOCUS ○ Full Body ○ Upper Body ○ Core ○ Lower Body ○ Active Rest

SAT

FOCUS ○ Full Body ○ Upper Body ○ Core ○ Lower Body ○ Active Rest

SUN

FOCUS ○ Full Body ○ Upper Body ○ Core ○ Lower Body ○ Active Rest

WORKOUT LOG

DATE				
WEIGHT				
SLEEP				
CALORIES				
WATER				

CORE EXERCISES	WEIGHT	REPS	WEIGHT	REPS	WEIGHT	REPS

UPPER BODY EXERCISES	WEIGHT	REPS	WEIGHT	REPS	WEIGHT	REPS

LOWER BODY EXERCISES	WEIGHT	REPS	WEIGHT	REPS	WEIGHT	REPS

CARDIO	TIME	DISTANCE	INTENSITY

WORKOUT LOG

DATE				
WEIGHT				
SLEEP				
CALORIES				
WATER				

CORE EXERCISES	WEIGHT	REPS	WEIGHT	REPS	WEIGHT	REPS

UPPER BODY EXERCISES	WEIGHT	REPS	WEIGHT	REPS	WEIGHT	REPS

LOWER BODY EXERCISES	WEIGHT	REPS	WEIGHT	REPS	WEIGHT	REPS

CARDIO	TIME	DISTANCE	INTENSITY

BEGINNER'S

Workout

WEEKLY PLANNER

Week 1

MONDAY _____   COMPLETED: YES / NO

MY FOCUS TODAY	WRITE 3 AFFIRMATIONS

WARM UP	WORKOUT	COOL DOWN

MOOD TRACKER

WATER TRACKER

TUESDAY _____   COMPLETED: YES / NO

MY FOCUS TODAY	WRITE 3 AFFIRMATIONS

WARM UP	WORKOUT	COOL DOWN

MOOD TRACKER

WATER TRACKER

WEDNESDAY _____   COMPLETED: YES / NO

MY FOCUS TODAY	WRITE 3 AFFIRMATIONS

WARM UP	WORKOUT	COOL DOWN

MOOD TRACKER

WATER TRACKER

Week 1

THURSDAY _____   COMPLETED: YES / NO

MY FOCUS TODAY	WRITE 3 AFFIRMATIONS

WARM UP	WORKOUT	COOL DOWN

MOOD TRACKER

WATER TRACKER

FRIDAY _____   COMPLETED: YES / NO

MY FOCUS TODAY	WRITE 3 AFFIRMATIONS

WARM UP	WORKOUT	COOL DOWN

MOOD TRACKER

WATER TRACKER

SATURDAY REST

SUNDAY _____   COMPLETED: YES / NO

SMALL STRETCH / WORKOUT	YOUR CHEAT FOOD REQUEST

You made it to first week! Good job.

Week 2

MONDAY _____

COMPLETED: YES / NO

MY FOCUS TODAY

WRITE 3 AFFIRMATIONS

WARM UP

WORKOUT

COOL DOWN

MOOD TRACKER

WATER TRACKER

TUESDAY _____

COMPLETED: YES / NO

MY FOCUS TODAY

WRITE 3 AFFIRMATIONS

WARM UP

WORKOUT

COOL DOWN

MOOD TRACKER

WATER TRACKER

WEDNESDAY _____

COMPLETED: YES / NO

MY FOCUS TODAY

WRITE 3 AFFIRMATIONS

WARM UP

WORKOUT

COOL DOWN

MOOD TRACKER

WATER TRACKER

Week 2

THURSDAY _____

COMPLETED: YES / NO

MY FOCUS TODAY	WRITE 3 AFFIRMATIONS

WARM UP	WORKOUT	COOL DOWN

MOOD TRACKER

WATER TRACKER

FRIDAY _____

COMPLETED: YES / NO

MY FOCUS TODAY	WRITE 3 AFFIRMATIONS

WARM UP	WORKOUT	COOL DOWN

MOOD TRACKER

WATER TRACKER

SATURDAY REST

SUNDAY _____

COMPLETED: YES / NO

SMALL STRETCH / WORKOUT	YOUR CHEAT FOOD REQUEST

You made it to second week! Good job.

Week 3

MONDAY _____

COMPLETED: YES / NO

MY FOCUS TODAY	WRITE 3 AFFIRMATIONS

WARM UP	WORKOUT	COOL DOWN

MOOD TRACKER

WATER TRACKER

TUESDAY _____

COMPLETED: YES / NO

MY FOCUS TODAY	WRITE 3 AFFIRMATIONS

WARM UP	WORKOUT	COOL DOWN

MOOD TRACKER

WATER TRACKER

WEDNESDAY _____

COMPLETED: YES / NO

MY FOCUS TODAY	WRITE 3 AFFIRMATIONS

WARM UP	WORKOUT	COOL DOWN

MOOD TRACKER

WATER TRACKER

Week 3

THURSDAY _____   COMPLETED: YES / NO

MY FOCUS TODAY	WRITE 3 AFFIRMATIONS

WARM UP	WORKOUT	COOL DOWN

MOOD TRACKER

WATER TRACKER

FRIDAY _____   COMPLETED: YES / NO

MY FOCUS TODAY	WRITE 3 AFFIRMATIONS

WARM UP	WORKOUT	COOL DOWN

MOOD TRACKER

WATER TRACKER

SATURDAY REST

SUNDAY _____   COMPLETED: YES / NO

SMALL STRETCH / WORKOUT	YOUR CHEAT FOOD REQUEST

You made it to third week! Good job.

Week 4

MONDAY _____ COMPLETED: YES / NO

MY FOCUS TODAY	WRITE 3 AFFIRMATIONS

WARM UP	WORKOUT	COOL DOWN

MOOD TRACKER

WATER TRACKER

TUESDAY _____ COMPLETED: YES / NO

MY FOCUS TODAY	WRITE 3 AFFIRMATIONS

WARM UP	WORKOUT	COOL DOWN

MOOD TRACKER

WATER TRACKER

WEDNESDAY _____ COMPLETED: YES / NO

MY FOCUS TODAY	WRITE 3 AFFIRMATIONS

WARM UP	WORKOUT	COOL DOWN

MOOD TRACKER

WATER TRACKER

Week 4

THURSDAY _____ COMPLETED: YES / NO

MY FOCUS TODAY	WRITE 3 AFFIRMATIONS

WARM UP	WORKOUT	COOL DOWN

MOOD TRACKER

WATER TRACKER

FRIDAY _____ COMPLETED: YES / NO

MY FOCUS TODAY	WRITE 3 AFFIRMATIONS

WARM UP	WORKOUT	COOL DOWN

MOOD TRACKER

WATER TRACKER

SATURDAY REST

SUNDAY _____ COMPLETED: YES / NO

SMALL STRETCH / WORKOUT	YOUR CHEAT FOOD REQUEST

You made it to forth week! Good job.

CHAPTER 12 - CONCLUSION – STAY MOTIVATED

Remember, the path to a stronger, healthier you isn't a sprint, it's a beautiful adventure. There will be days when your muscles ache, your breath won't cooperate, and your mind whispers doubts. But don't let those whispers win.

Instead, hold onto the reason you started. Picture the joy of movement, the confidence of a stronger body, the peace of a calmer mind. Let those visions fuel your fire, guide your steps, and remind you why this journey is worth every bead of sweat, every ache, every moment of dedication.

Celebrate your victories, big and small. Did you hold that pose a little longer? Did you climb that hill without stopping? Did you wake up feeling energized and ready to move? These are the milestones that truly matter, the whispers of your body and spirit telling you you're on the right track.

Find your tribe, your community of fellow travelers on this path. Share your struggles, celebrate your triumphs, and lean on each other for support. Together, you can inspire, motivate, and remind each other that you're not alone.

And most importantly, be kind to yourself. This journey is yours, unique and ever-evolving. There will be detours, setbacks, and days when you just need to rest. Allow yourself the grace to be human, to stumble, and then rise again, stronger and more determined than before.

Remember, motivation isn't a fleeting spark, it's a burning ember you tend to with every mindful breath, every intentional movement, every small step forward. So, keep tending that ember, keep believing in yourself, and keep moving. The best version of you is waiting just beyond the next bend, and the journey itself is the greatest reward.

Now, let's share the spark! If this book has resonated with you, consider leaving a positive review. Your words can ignite the flame of motivation in others, inspiring them to embark on their own transformative journeys.

And think of the gift of well-being! This book can be a beautiful present for loved ones, friends, and family. Share the power of movement, the joy of self-discovery, and the gift of a stronger, healthier them.

Let's move with joy, breathe with purpose, and conquer this adventure together, one mindful step at a time. You've got this! And remember, you're not alone. We're all on this journey, cheering each other on, one positive review and shared gift at a time.

Now go forth, spread the word, and let the movement begin!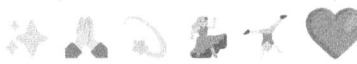

LEGAL DETAILS

Before embarking on this transformative 28-day wall Pilates journey, it's essential to understand some legal aspects that ensure a safe and enjoyable experience. The information provided in this book is intended for general informational purposes only. It does not replace professional medical advice, diagnosis, or treatment.

Consult with a qualified healthcare professional before beginning any new exercise program, especially if you have pre-existing health conditions or concerns. The exercises and practices outlined in this book may not be suitable for everyone, and individual circumstances should be taken into account.

The author and publisher of this book are not responsible for any injuries or health issues that may result from the use of the information contained herein. It is crucial to listen to your body, modify exercises as needed, and prioritize safety during your Pilates practice.

Respect copyright and intellectual property rights. The content, including text and illustrations, is protected by copyright law. Reproduction, distribution, or unauthorized use of any part of this book without permission is prohibited.

By engaging in the Pilates workouts and following the guidelines in this book, you acknowledge and agree to the terms outlined here. Remember, your health and safety are the top priorities. If you have any questions or concerns about the information presented, seek professional advice to ensure your fitness journey is tailored to your individual needs.